Digital Skills for Nursing Studies and Practice

Sara Miller McCune founded SAGE Publishing in 1965 to support the dissemination of usable knowledge and educate a global community. SAGE publishes more than 1000 journals and over 800 new books each year, spanning a wide range of subject areas. Our growing selection of library products includes archives, data, case studies and video. SAGE remains majority owned by our founder and after her lifetime will become owned by a charitable trust that secures the company's continued independence.

Los Angeles | London | New Delhi | Singapore | Washington DC | Melbourne

Digital Skills for Nursing Studies and Practice

Edited by
Cristina M. Vasilica
Emma Gillaspy
Neil Withnell

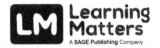

Learning Matters
A SAGE Publishing Company
1 Oliver's Yard
55 City Road
London EC1Y 1SP

SAGE Publications Inc.
2455 Teller Road
Thousand Oaks, California 91320

SAGE Publications India Pvt Ltd
B 1/I 1 Mohan Cooperative Industrial Area
Mathura Road
New Delhi 110 044

SAGE Publications Asia-Pacific Pte Ltd
3 Church Street
#10-04 Samsung Hub
Singapore 049483

Editor: Martha Cunneen
Development editor: Sarah Turpie
Senior project editor: Chris Marke
Marketing manager: Ruslana Khatagova
Cover design: Sheila Tong
Typeset by: C&M Digitals (P) Ltd, Chennai, India
Printed in the UK

Library of Congress Control Number: 2022951759

British Library Cataloguing in Publication Data

A catalogue record for this book is available from the British Library

ISBN 978-1-5297-9192-1
ISBN 978-1-5297-9191-4 (pbk)

At SAGE we take sustainability seriously. Most of our products are printed in the UK using responsibly sourced papers and boards. When we print overseas we ensure sustainable papers are used as measured by the PREPS grading system. We undertake an annual audit to monitor our sustainability.

Contents

TRANSFORMING NURSING PRACTICE

Transforming Nursing Practice is a series tailor made for pre-registration student nurses. Each book in the series is:

- Affordable
- Mapped to the NMC Standards of proficiency for registered nurses
- Full of active learning features
- Focused on applying theory to practice

Each book addresses a core topic and they have been carefully developed to be simple to use, quick to read and written in clear language.

An invaluable series of books that explicitly relates to the NMC standards. Each book covers a different topic that students need to explore in order to develop into a qualified nurse... I would recommend this series to all Pre-Registered nursing students whatever their field or year of study.

LINDA ROBSON,
Senior Lecturer at Edge Hill University

Many titles in the series are on our recommended reading list and for good reason - the content is up to date and easy to read. These are the books that actually get used beyond training and into your nursing career.

EMMA LYDON,
Adult Student Nursing

ABOUT THE SERIES EDITORS

DR MOOI STANDING is an Independent Nursing Consultant (UK and International) and is responsible for the core knowledge, adult nursing and personal and professional learning skills titles. She is an experienced NMC Quality Assurance Reviewer of educational programmes and a Professional Regulator Panellist on the NMC Practice Committee. Mooi is also Board member of Special Olympics Malaysia, enabling people with intellectual disabilities to participate in sports and athletics nationally and internationally.

DR SANDRA WALKER is a Clinical Academic in Mental Health working between Southern Health Trust and the University of Southampton and responsible for the mental health nursing titles. She is a Qualified Mental Health Nurse with a wide range of clinical experience spanning more than 25 years.

BESTSELLING TEXTBOOKS

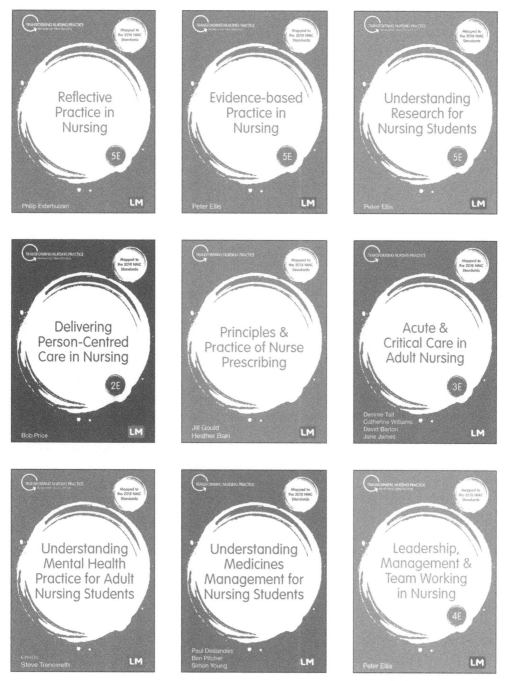

You can find a full list of textbooks in the *Transforming Nursing Practice* series at
https://uk.sagepub.com/TNP-series

About the Authors

Dilla Davis from the University of Salford is a lecturer in adult nursing, programme lead for MSc Diabetes Care and MSc in Leadership in Education. @dilla_davis

Janet Garner from the Comensus group at the University of Central Lancashire is a staff facilitator for the School of Nursing. @UCLanComensus @JMGarner5

Lisa Garwood-Cross is a Research Fellow at the University of Salford. Lisa's work relates to the intersections of digital technology, social media and digital health. @lgarwood-cross

Kirstie Harrison is a Lecturer in Pre-Registration Nursing and one of the School of Nursing's Active Blended Learning Leads at the University of Central Lancashire. @Kirstie130.

Michael Haslam from The University of Central Lancashire is a Senior Lecturer in Mental Health Nursing. @mbhaslam

Steph Holmes from the Comensus group at the University of Central Lancashire is a volunteer community member, facilitator of Chrysalis Transsexual Support Groups and governor of Lancashire and South Cumbria NHS Foundation Trust. @ChrysalisTSG

Amanda Miller from Edge Hill University is the Head of Simulation and Skills and Senior Learning and Teaching Fellow (Simulation). @AJMillerSim

Yeliz Prior from the University of Salford is a Professor of Clinical Rehabilitation at the University of Salford and Programme Lead for the Centre for Doctoral Training in Prosthetics and Orthotics. @ProfYelizPrior

Mike Smith is a Lecturer in Mental Health Nursing and one of the School of Nursing's Active Blended Learning Leads at the University of Central Lancashire. @MikeSmithMHN

Nicky Varley is a Lecturer in Children and Young People's Nursing and one of the School of Nursing's Active Blended Learning Leads at the University of Central Lancashire. @Nickyvar

Matthew Wynn from the University of Salford is a lecturer in adult nursing, a researcher in digital health and honorary tissue viability specialist nurse. @MatthewWynn96

Dr Cristina M. Vasilica (lead editor and author)

Cristina is a Reader in Digital Health and Head of Digital Education at the University of Salford. With a background in digital business, Cristina worked in the industry before joining Academia. Passionate about technology and its ability to empower social mobility, innovation and impact, Cristina has worked towards becoming a recognised international leader in digital health. Her current work is organised into three intertwined workstreams – digital engagement, digital methods and digital education – spanning across disciplines to make more effective use of resources, strengthen impact and long-term sustainability in digital health. Cristina has a significant track record of translating research into teaching and learning. She introduced the University of Salford Digital Skills Passport (DiSkPass^{TM}) for the nursing curriculum, which aims to equip all nursing students with digital capabilities required for the digitisation of care provision. @cristinavas

Dr Emma Gillaspy (editor and author)

Emma is a Reader in Creative and Collaborative Learning at the University of Central Lancashire. Emma is a National Teaching Fellow, #creativeHE host, academic developer and executive coach. Emma activates the passions of learners and empowers them to reach their potential through a unique blend of appreciative enquiry-based coaching, heutagogy and social learning. Emma uses creative materials and non-linear digital technologies to support this approach which enables non-verbal ways of knowing to emerge, leading to congruent development aligned with learners' core values and beliefs. @egillaspy

Neil Withnell (editor and author)

A registered mental health nurse, Neil joined the University of Salford in July 2002 as a Lecturer Practitioner in Mental Health Nursing. He made the move to become a full-time Lecturer in November 2003 and has carried out various roles before his current role as Associate Dean Academic Student Experience. Neil is passionate about enhancing the student experience and has a keen interest in social media, flexible learning, creative education and technology-enhanced learning. @neilwithnell

With the growth of technology and the rapid uptake of digital innovations in healthcare, it is only logical for us as student nurses to become familiar with and proficient in digital skills. This book perfectly summarises the importance of the digital world, how it supports nursing practice, its potential and how we as professionals can use it safely and effectively. I think it is an essential asset for every student nurse's bookshelf!

Karolina Staniecka @karolinaviolet, student nurse, University of Salford

Introduction

About this book

Digital Skills for Nursing Studies and Practice is a comprehensive text for anyone studying or working in the nursing profession wanting to assess and develop their digital capabilities.

The book will cover the basics of what digital capabilities are and why they are needed. It explores technical and functional capabilities, including digital devices, data, communication, creation, collaboration, curation and digital innovation. Given the increased use of digital technologies, tools and advice on digital well-being and staying safe online are provided. In summary, the book will equip nursing students and trainee nursing associates with the digital mindset they will need to succeed in their studies and future career. We also expect other health and social care students and professionals to find the book useful and relevant.

The book is intended to be read either as a whole or in small sections dependent on the need of the reader. An initial self-assessment will help the reader follow specific areas of interest. The book draws upon student and patient insights, case scenarios and interactive activities that encourage readers to reflect on and apply their learning.

Why Digital Skills?

The title of the book is designed to address the future nursing workforce that needs to be ready for an ever-changing landscape and work in a digitally enabled sector. The term 'digital skills' is used as a broader approach that encapsulates digital capabilities and digital literacies, including knowledge on how to remain at the forefront of digital advancements in healthcare. It responds to current societal and political drivers that recommend the appropriate level of digital literacy training for healthcare students.

Book structure

Chapter 1: Why digital capabilities are essential for nurses

Digital skills and capabilities have become a key skill required for health students and the healthcare workforce. According to the European Commission, all jobs require digital skills; it is envisaged that almost all healthcare jobs will require fundamental digital capabilities (communication, participation, information searching, data management, etc.).

This opening chapter provides an overview of digital skills and capabilities required to thrive in the digital economy. Setting the scene for the book, the chapter covers definitions, application and impact. The chapter concludes with a self-assessment so that readers can appreciate their current position and determine their developmental needs.

Chapter 2: Digital toolkit: devices, platforms and tools to support your practice

This focuses on digital devices and digital platforms which are redefining relationships in this hyperactive and hyperconnected world. There are a multitude of digital devices that offer a variety of functionalities and uses. The benefits and limitations of a variety of devices and platforms with benefits and limitations/challenges are discussed in this chapter. The chapter highlights applications to nursing studies and practice as well as relevance to patient outcomes and innovation.

Chapter 3: Looking after the digital well-being of yourself and others

Two aspects of digital well-being are explored in this chapter – using digital devices to improve health and well-being; and maintaining a healthy relationship with technology. As health professionals, it is important to understand the utility of technology to improve outcomes for patients and the public. Similarly, these concepts are important at a personal level to safely participate in online communities and networks, act in accordance with the nursing code of practice, establish norms, negotiate conflict, manage digital workload and overall be in a safe online space, in that personal growth is possible.

Chapter 4: Harnessing the potential of your digital collaborations

Living in a digital society encompasses the need to work together in virtual spaces for the benefit of others, particularly for our service users and for our own personal development. A myriad of devices and platforms are discussed in this chapter which enable increased collaboration between individuals and the care team, contributing to positive health outcomes. Digital collaboration remains an important aspect of personal development through shared knowledge, feedback, access to information and better information workflows. This chapter explores the benefits and challenges of a wide range of collaboration tools and practices.

Chapter 5: Unleashing your digital creativity to enhance person-centred care

User generated content is fundamental to the sustainability of digital and social platforms. This chapter explores the creation and co-creation of digital content for service users, carers, patients and families. The authors consider the impact that digital technology has had on health and social care communication and the nursing profession. Barriers to digital engagement for patients and families are explored and the reader is encouraged to harness their creative ideas for the benefit of all.

Chapter 6: Digital curation: implications for the nursing student and nursing practice

The proliferation of the social web has allowed people to engage in the user-generated content process and has created a massive volume of information by members of the public, yet organisations are still sceptical to utilise it. Questions such as 'is the information trustworthy, real, valuable, credible' remain. Another challenge associated with this phenomenon is being able to navigate through the volume of information shared. In this chapter, curation tools and processes are discussed to equip the reader with knowledge on how to curate effectively. The chapter explores the opportunities for co-curation with a range of people, including peers, patients, families and carers.

Chapter 7: Digital innovation in healthcare

This chapter discusses the evidence base for digital innovations that have driven improvements in health and social care. The impact of these innovations on nursing practice are explored through a variety of case studies and activities. The reader is encouraged to consider the digital capabilities needed to find and evaluate relevant evidence, novel digital approaches used in research to collect and access data, and digital methods. The chapter enhances the reader's understanding of the ethical challenges associated with digital technologies, information and clinical data in e-research.

Chapter 8: Your ongoing digital development

This chapter summarises the key learning points across all of the chapters in the book. Adopting a reflective style, readers are encouraged to identify what they have learnt from their explorations in each chapter and how this contributes to their professional identity as nurses. Using the common solutions-focused coaching model *OSKAR*, the reader identifies personal *objectives* for the development of their digital capabilities in relation to their future nursing practice and *scores* their current practice in each key area of digital capability. The reader considers what *knowledge*, skills or resources they need to successfully reach their goals. Through a process of *affirmation*, the reader reflects on their strengths and how these can be leveraged to take positive actions towards their goal. Finally, the reader is encouraged to identify measures to *review* their ongoing progress and consider how this will impact on their professional development as a digitally enabled nurse.

Mapping to the Health and Care Digital Capability Framework

Requirements for the NMC Standards of Proficiency for Registered Nurses are considered within the book, and all chapters are mapped to the Health and Care Digital Capability Framework (Health Education England, 2018). The framework includes six domains and progression through four different levels of digital capability. Each chapter is mapped against specific domains, providing the learner with a level 2 in digital capability. We believe that level 2 equips the learner with fundamental skills required to perform well in a digitally enabled environment.

Learning features

Learning from reading text is not always easy. Therefore, to provide variety and to assist with the development of independent learning skills and the application of theory to practice, this book contains activities, case studies, scenarios, useful websites and other materials to enable you to participate in your own learning. You will need to develop your own study skills and 'learn how to learn' to get the best from the material. The book cannot provide all the answers, but instead provides a framework for your learning.

The activities in the book will help you to make sense of, and learn about, the material being presented. Some activities ask you to reflect on aspects of practice, or your experience of it, or the people or situations you encounter. Reflection is an essential skill in nursing, and it helps you to understand the world around you and often to identify how things might be improved. Other activities will help you develop key graduate skills such as your ability to think critically about a topic in order to challenge assumptions, or your ability to research a topic and find appropriate information and evidence, and to be able to make decisions using that evidence in situations that are often difficult and time-pressured.

All the activities require you to take a break from reading the text, think through the issues presented and carry out some independent study, possibly using the internet. Where appropriate, there are sample answers presented at the end of each chapter, and these will help you to understand more fully your own reflections and independent study. Remember, academic study will always require independent work; attending classes at university will never be enough to be successful on your programme, and these activities will help to deepen your knowledge and understanding of the issues under scrutiny and give you practice at working on your own.

You might want to think about completing these activities as part of your personal development plan (PDP) or portfolio. After completing each activity, write it up in your PDP or portfolio in a section devoted to that particular skill, then look back over time to see how far you are developing. You can also do more of the activities for an area that you have identified a weakness in, which will help build your skill and confidence in this area.

You will find the Twitter handles of all the authors in their biographies. Do connect with us if you have any questions or comments about the topics in this book. We hope you enjoy this book. Remember, 'every nurse is an e-nurse' and good luck with your studies!

Chapter 1 Why digital capabilities are essential for nurses

Cristina M. Vasilica and Neil Withnell

with contributions from Rob Finnigan

HEE Digital Capabilities Framework

This book is intended to be used by student and registered nurses, and those supporting them to improve digital competencies. It is shaped using the Health and Care Digital Capability Framework (Figure 1.1).

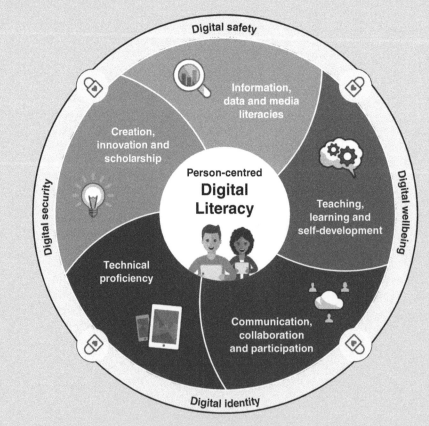

Figure 1.1 Health and Care Digital Capability Framework (Health Education England, 2018)

The framework includes six domains, and progression through four different levels of digital capability. Each chapter is mapped against specific domains, providing the learner with a level 2 in digital capability. We believe that level 2 equips the learner with fundamental skills required to perform well in a digitally enabled environment.

Chapter aims

After reading this chapter, you will be able to:

- understand the importance of digital skills as an integral subset of digital health transformation;
- gain knowledge of digital skills, developmental frameworks and relevance to nursing practice;
- assess your own capabilities using a self-assessment tool.

Introduction

I appreciate how much the use of social media, digital skills, digital technologies and its use in communication and information sharing can all have positive health outcomes for those people who engage with it.

(Student nurse)

Digital skills are now an essential part of daily activities from social interaction to shopping, paying bills, banking and accessing information. The use of various platforms enables us to go about our daily life with everything we need at our fingertips. Modern workplaces and educational settings encourage and support people to engage in digital practices.

In our work with health students and the healthcare workforce, we recognised that digital skills and capabilities have become a key skill required to achieve digital transformation and improve practice. Digital health refers to the use of technology in areas such as eHealth, mHealth, health informatics, telehealth, wearable devices, Internet of Things and medical devices applied to health (Brice and Almond, 2020). It represents an evolutionary adaptation of the art and science of medicine to pervasive information and communication technologies (ICTs). A classification of digital health interventions (DHIs) categories has been compiled by the World Health Organization (WHO), in an attempt to create a shared language describing the different ways in which digital technology is used in health (World Health Organization, 2021).

It is envisaged that almost all healthcare jobs, including nursing, will require fundamental digital capabilities that will support communication, participation, information search, data management and innovation. The recent Coronavirus (COVID-19) pandemic, which placed unprecedented demands on the health service systems and forced changes in practice, highlighted the importance of being a digital nurse practitioner. Embracing the changes and being at the forefront of digital innovation will bring a competitive edge to nursing education.

This opening chapter provides an overview of digital skills and capabilities required for nurses to become a digital nurse professional and thrive in the digital economy. Setting the scene for the book, the chapter covers definitions, developmental frameworks and the importance of digital skills for nursing education and practice. The chapter concludes with a self-assessment so that the readers can appreciate their current position and determine their developmental needs.

Digital technology and the paradigm shift in nursing practice capabilities

In the twenty-first century, it is recognised that 'digital' has changed the way that we work, live and function. This is recognised at a global level, within the sphere of digital health. In 2020, the WHO, drawing on its previous resolutions on digital health, adopted a global strategy on digital health to strengthen the health system using digital technologies (World Health Organization, 2021) and to achieve a global vision promoting global collaboration and knowledge sharing in the field (Mariano, 2020). The principles indicate that all countries should:

1. commit to developments;
2. create a robust strategy for digital ecosystems that considers leadership, financial, organisational, human and technological resources;
3. strengthen governance, promote appropriate and safe use of technology, and
4. support the needs of less-developed countries in implementing digital health technologies.

(World Health Organization, 2021)

The European Commission also aims to offer access to safe digital services in health, and has established three top priorities:

1. Safe access to health data across borders.
2. Working across the EU to share information and expertise to create personalised medicine.

3. Person-centred care through citizen empowerment, feedback and access to digital tools.

(European Commission, 2018)

This vision can be achieved with a safe, trusted and collaborative digital health eco-system, according to the latest report from Digital Europe. This means having an electronic healthcare record available in all EU countries. For this to be possible, the report emphasises four pillars required to achieve trust in the system and support data sharing, including demonstrating benefits for all communities, security by design, leverage existing health-data success and increasing digital literacy (DigitalEurope, 2021). Notably, digital skills are an essential success factor in achieving digital health.

In the United Kingdom, the NHS is also undergoing a digital transformation as technology advances and healthcare consumers seek novel, digitally driven ways of receiving care. The NHS Long Term Plan (2019) places great emphasis on the future of digitally enabled care, highlighting that it will become mainstream across the NHS. The time for action to embed data and digital technology within the NHS to address unprecedented demands and pressures imposed by the pandemic is 'now' according to a report by the Department of Health and Social Care published in 2021. The report further acknowledges that a mindset is required to achieve the digital transformation and makes recommendations for practice. A key recommendation is that NHS clinicians are required to understand the importance of data and the digital in order to effectively use it as part of their practice (Department of Health and Social Care, 2021). The paradigm shift towards digital capabilities and values required to deliver care was previously reinforced by Erick Topol, who touches upon the need to develop understanding of digital health technologies and build digital skills among the healthcare workforce (Topol Review, 2019). This is further articulated in the Royal College of Nursing vision of a digital enabled workplace, in that every nurse should thrive to be an 'e-nurse' by 2020 (Royal College of Nursing, 2018). Health Education England is leading on the work to operationalise this 'e-nurse' or 'digital healthcare professional' vision through digital skills training and a developmental framework. Other streams of work were implemented to develop digital leaders; NHS Digital Academy was launched in 2017 and continues to support the development of digital leaders through a Digital Health Leadership programme (NHS Digital Academy, 2021).

This whole paradigm shift is not just specific to leaders and governmental strategists. People are wanting better quality healthcare, and by enabling everyone to have more autonomy and empowerment in their healthcare, this greatly enhances patient care.

It is therefore paramount that anyone working and learning in healthcare needs to have digital skills and capabilities to be able to provide the best possible care to all. Provision of digital capabilities should form an integral part of nursing training and continue into the nursing profession. In a previous study, we asked our nursing students to reflect on the importance of digital skills and digital health training and they identified the following key aspects: 'opened me up to new ideas'; 'be at the forefront of the technological revolution'; 'keep up-to-date with technology and training'.

They also referred to the need to change training and current policy to reflect the digital innovations:

> *Training will be needed to bring healthcare together in a new digital era.*
>
> *The code . . . will need to change to incorporate a nurses digital self.*

> (Gillaspy and Vasilica, 2021)

We asked 30 nurses why digital skills are important to them. The key aspects in their response include communication, collaboration and safety (Figure 1.2).

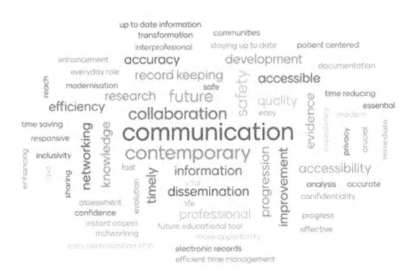

Figure 1.2 Nurses' perceptions of the importance of digital skills

Digital health: a patient's perspective

Digital technologies bring a new dimension to patients' engagement with their health. Rob Finnigan, a patient managing a long-term condition, shared his experiences and the impact of using digital technologies:

> *My kidneys failed in 2002 due to an inherited condition and I'm now in my 19th year post-transplant.*
>
> *When I was initially diagnosed with kidney failure, the news was overwhelming, Although I attended many GP appointments, I didn't engage at all with the prospect*

of my kidneys failing, I was focused solely on my young family, my burgeoning career and our chunky mortgage. As a consequence of my approach, I was given 20 minutes to decide which treatment modality I wanted to follow.

I opted to dialyse at home in the hope that it would allow me to carry on working and, thankfully, I had a supportive employer at the time. While my approach allowed me to carry on working, it's fair to say dialysis was simply a process I followed and not something I fully understood.

Luckily, I received a kidney 11 months later and dialysis became a thing of the past although, despite my transplant, I never felt in control. The issues I encountered felt largely beyond my control and understanding. This absence of control is a frequent, non-clinical side effect of a chronic illness diagnosis and while I carried on working, many in a similar position found they were unable to work, further exacerbating the lack of control which was compounded by financial and psychosocial issues.

My sense of control only increased when I registered to use an online portal, PatientView (it later became an app) which not only allowed me to see my blood tests results within 24 hours of the tests, but also gave me an explanation of every aspect of my blood chemistry. This was revelatory. Now I was able to drive the conversation with my consultant. If something in my blood results appeared abnormal, I could contact the transplant team at my renal centre before they did their multidisciplinary assessment.

This newfound resource, along with a few other things such as supporting other patients in closed Facebook groups (Kidney Information Network), changed my life. In my mid-50s I had resigned myself to not working again, but I gained a position as a Patient Advocacy Officer with Kidney Care UK purely because my self-confidence and self-esteem had been lifted by my increased sense of control and understanding.

Sadly, PatientView was poorly promoted within the renal community, each renal centre administered it differently and many failed to use all its functionality. I suspect some clinicians failed to support the promotion of PatientView because they failed to see how the information it provided could be of benefit to patients; they perceived the information to be of value to them alone.

PatientView is closing down to be replaced by the Patients Know Best platform, but I fear the same mistakes of poor promotion will be repeated. We need to ensure that every patient with access to these resources understands how the information can help them individually to increase their sense of control, enhance their understanding and, potentially, improve their outcomes. It is my belief that patient mentors are best placed to increase the use of such platforms.

Rob's experiences highlight the potential positive impact of digital technology, from health to social outcomes. It facilitates a greater self-management of his health and well-being, and supports his return to full-time employment.

Activity 1.1   Reflection

Reflect on Rob's experiences of PatientView (now replaced with Patients Know Best) and identify three aspects that you would have changed in promoting the platform to patients and the key skills that you would need to achieve that.

As this activity is based on your own reflection, no answer is given at the end of this chapter.

The benefits and challenges of incorporating digital technology into nursing practice

Incorporating digital skills, capabilities and technologies into healthcare has many benefits and challenges – both for nurses and patients. The evidence collated in Table 1.1 presents a snapshot of benefits and challenges for your practice, alongside examples of technologies; more depth is provided in subsequent chapters.

Digital skills: a myriad of terms and developmental frameworks

A multitude of terms are used to encompass the 'skills' necessary to work and live in a digitally driven society. Over the years, the approach to define digital skills transcended from a technical orientation towards a broader perspective (capabilities) that embodies content related and higher order cognitive abilities, behaviour and culture (Claro et al., 2012; van Laar et al., 2020).

The discourse around digital skills, despite its current prominence, has been around for decades. During the 1990s, with the widespread use of the internet, the term 'computer literacy' was used to highlight the social implications of technology (Tuman, 1992). In 2003, the UK government recognised the importance of information and communication technology (ICT) as a twenty-first-century skill, and introduced it as a core skill to complement literacy and numeracy skills (Department for Education and Skills, 2003). Researchers have proposed different practical and developmental frameworks to inform training and development; a snapshot is presented in Table 1.2. While the application of digital skills varies across sectors (Kispeter, 2018), the fundamental skills and competencies required are similar, as highlighted in Table 1.2. For example, communication is a competency identified in all frameworks.

Benefits	Challenges	Example of digital health technologies
Patients		
• Patient-centred care • Self-management of long-term conditions • Empowerment • Treatment compliance • Reliable and fast access to services	• Health literacy and digital capability • Access to infrastructure (platforms, internet, devices) • Usability of platform (poor system design) • Plain language • Decline in the therapeutic relationship	• Telehealth solutions (e.g., video conferencing solutions) • Mobile health (apps) (e.g., NHS app) • Personal health records • Social media
Access to health and well-being information	• Information reliability and accuracy • Readable and easy to comprehend	• Social media platforms • Internet searches • Apps
Reduced isolation through peer support	• Inappropriate behaviour • Moderation	• Social media groups • Forums • Chatrooms
Nurses		
Benefits for health and care system • High-quality care through enhanced patient monitoring and data that can inform personalised care pathways • Increase efficiency of care by removing the time needed to wade through paperwork • Cost-effective and convenient care solutions • Reduce medication errors	• Digital capabilities • Documentation quality concerns • Data accuracy • Errors (human/technology) • Algorithm bias and reliability on existing data (which can be inconsistent)	• EPR systems • Artificial Intelligence • ePrescribing systems
Personal development • Access to information • Networking and communication • Learning and ongoing personal development	• Access, cost of development and maintenance of training solution	• Social media, forums • Cross Reality (Virtual Reality, Augmented Reality, Mixed Reality) • Digital learning (e-learning)

Table 1.1   The benefits and challenges of digital technology

Framework	Domains				
General frameworks					
DigComp Framework (European Union) (Carretero et al., 2017), proficiency: 'foundation' to 'highly specialised'					
Communication and collaboration	Information and data literacy	Digital content creation	Problem solving	Safety	
Essential Digital Skills Framework (Department for Education, 2018)					
Communicating	Handling information and content	Transacting	Problem solving	Being safe and legal online	
JISC Digital Capabilities Framework (JISC, 2015), proficiency levels: developing, capable or proficient					
Digital collaboration, communication and participation	Information, data and media literacy	Digital creation, problem solving and innovation	ICT proficiency	Digital identity and well-being	Digital learning and development
Health and nursing-specific competency frameworks					
Health and Care Digital Capabilities Framework (2018) (HEE, 2018). Proficiency levels: level 1 – aware; level 2 – able; level 3 – capable; level 4 – expert.					
Communication, collaboration and participation	Information, data and content	Creation, innovation and research	Technical proficiency	Digital identity, well-being, safety and security	Teaching, learning and self-development
Core competencies required for nursing telehealth (core skills) (van Houwelingen et al., 2016)					
Communication skills	Coaching skills	Combine clinical experience with telehealth	Clinical knowledge	Ethical awareness	Supportive attitude

Table 1.2 A snapshot of Digital Skills Frameworks

The most prevalent proficiencies, recognised in the majority of frameworks are:

- functional skills (ICT or technical skills);
- digital communication, collaboration and participation in digital spaces;
- online safety, security and ethics;
- information, data and content;
- creation, research and innovation.

Other fundamental skills allowing continuous self-development are problem solving, critical thinking and understanding the impact of being digitally capable for you and the service users.

A more exhaustive list of frameworks focused on health and person-centred digital healthcare is provided by Brice and Almond (2020). An additional review highlights the extent to which digital capabilities are recognised at a strategic level (Nazeha et al., 2020). It identified 14 digital capabilities frameworks focused on nursing. Interestingly, a large number of frameworks are focused on health informatics (technology to organise health records) rather than digital health as a whole.

Terms such as 'digital healthcare professional', or 'e-nurse' allude to health professionals with skills required to be digitally competent (Brice and Almond, 2020; Royal College of Nursing, 2018). In 2018, Health Education England launched their 'Health and Care Digital Capability Framework' which is a developmental framework encouraging positive attitudes towards the digital (Health Education England, 2018). The framework encompasses six domains and progression through four different levels of digital capability. The following chapters include competencies related to each domain (see Table 1.3).

Chapter	Domain	
2	Information, data and content; Teaching, learning and self-development; Communication, collaboration and participation; Technical proficiency	
3	Digital identity, well-being, safety and security; Teaching, learning and self-development	
4	Communication, collaboration and participation; Information, data and content; Teaching, learning and self-development; Digital identity, well-being, safety and security	Problem solving, critical thinking and impact
5	Creation, innovation and research; Information, data and content; Teaching, learning and self-development; Communication, collaboration and participation; Technical proficiency; creation, innovation and research	
6	Communication, collaboration and participation; Creation, innovation and research; Information, data and content	
7	Creation, innovation and research; Information, data and content	
8	Teaching, learning and self-development	

Table 1.3 Mapping skills against the health and care digital capability framework

The majority of evidence in the field uses digital skills as a shorthand to competencies, capabilities, e-skills knowledge, behaviours, attitudes and character traits (Brice and Almond, 2020; Kispeter, 2018). This book uses digital skills and digital competencies synonymously.

Huhman (2011), a career manager expert, interpreted digital skills as the proficiency to use technology, and a positive mindset to navigate and apply the skills to context. Indeed, previous evidence confirms the assumption that acquiring technical skills will not suffice to empower health professionals to embrace technology (Brice and Almond, 2020). It draws attention to the complex human behaviour and relies on the intrinsic motivation to invest time and effort into gaining new knowledge. A variety of determinants influence twenty-first-century digital skills, thus including demographic, socioeconomic, personality, psychological, mental, motivational, social support, training and culture (van Laar et al., 2020).

Digital competence is recognised as 'T-shaped skill set' in that a basic knowledge about digital technologies is necessary with an in-depth knowledge of application in the particular area of practice (European Schoolnet, 2016). T-shaped skills for a student nurse (and a future nurse professional) are needed to navigate through change, largely driven by rapid technological changes of the healthcare field. For example, based on van Houwelingen et al. (2016) competencies for nursing telehealth activities, nurses require general knowledge about using telehealth systems alongside in-depth knowledge about organisational policy and protocols such as data governance, data protection, consent (aligns with 'Digital identity, well-being, safety and security', Health and Care Digital Capability Framework). In addition, knowledge of benefits, clinical limitations of technology and critical knowledge on how to collect health-related data to monitor patients is required (aligns with 'Information, data and content', Health and Care Digital Capability Framework).

A positive attitude for the provision of telehealth is also necessary, thus including professional integrity, honesty, empathy and friendliness, and overall supporting the patients, while enhancing their confidence and trust in technology.

Considering Rob's account of PatientView's implementation for renal patients, not all clinicians realised its benefits for patient-centred care, nor supported patients' engagement with the platform. Yet, patients who engaged with the platform highlighted high levels of user satisfaction with the service (Mukoro, 2012), findings that resonate with Rob's positive outcomes.

Despite the availability and increased use of online portals, their potential for self-management is not fully explored (Hazara et al., 2019). The study by Hazara and colleagues explored the perspective of inactive account holders and reported loss of login credentials and lack of awareness of whom to contact (Hazara et al., 2019). This highlights a lack of communication between patients and clinicians, supporting the need for communication competencies.

Ultimately, being digitally literate, means having the capability to use digital technologies to work in interdisciplinary teams, across different systems and cultures, as well as acquiring self-knowledge to provide the best possible care. It can enable faster access to reliable resources and networks, contributing to a more personalised, independent and self-determined learning pathway.

Activity 1.2   Your proficiency and goals

Being aware that your digital proficiencies allow you to set up goals and focus on specific development areas.

You can use specific tools to test your digital competencies. Below, we offer a series of digital systems that you can use.

a.   DigComp self-assessment (free to use). More information is available via the QR code below.

b.   The JISC discovery tool (available to staff and students from subscribing organisations only). Please check with your organisation if JISC is available. Use the QR code to navigate to the tool.

c.   Health Education England Digital Literacy Self-Assessment Diagnostic Tool

Designed for health professionals: the tool can be used to determine your current digital literacy levels and help identify areas of learning need. Please check with your institution if the tool is available. More information is available via the QR code below.

Use one of the digital tools (a–c) to self-assess your digital capabilities, identify strengths and opportunities for further personal development. Review the report and the domains (areas) in which you do well and not so well. How do you plan to develop your skills in the future? You might want to use the results to formulate your PDR goal and use the chapters to further your knowledge and skills.

As this activity is based on your own reflection, no answer is given at the end of the chapter.

The COVID-19 pandemic highlighted how technology can be used to address challenges within the healthcare systems and beyond. The pandemic has disrupted healthcare directly in addition to indirect effects posed by the mitigation efforts (e.g., reorganise care, face-to-face appointments, reorganise manpower). This triggered a renewed interest in digital health solutions, including telehealth (e.g., video consultations, monitoring tools, online information), AI systems (detection, diagnosis, epidemiological predictions and future forecasts) and IoT (home monitoring systems, including symptom data, pulse oximetry) (Greenhalgh et al., 2020; Oliver et al., 2022). Patients turned to social media to access information, peer support and keep up with the volatile situation.

The challenging period has also exposed the digital divide in education, healthcare staff and patients. The rapid move to online learning and services exposed a lack of digital capabilities, a woeful divide of those who had and those who didn't have access to technologies, fragile bandwidths and a total lack of preparedness. Without digital capabilities, technology has the potential to negatively affect nursing education in practice, increasing feelings of anxiety, disconnection and frustration, which ultimately can impact on practice.

Case study: Yolanda's digital context

Yolanda is a first-year student nurse, studying adult nursing. She gained a place on the programme having completed a BTEC and has previously worked as a bank nurse to gain some clinical experience. Yolanda herself states that she struggles with technology and tends to avoid using computers and smart devices, except to keep in touch with family and friends. She has considered an IT course, but has not taken this up, as she feels lacking in confidence.

Activity 1.3   Advise Yolanda

Considering Yolanda's digital context, outline five top tips to boost her confidence in taking up a course; consider what are her proficiency levels, what goals she can set up and why digital skills are important.

An outline answer is provided at the end of this chapter.

Chapter summary

This chapter has provided an introduction to digital capabilities within the context of health, further highlighting a paradigm shift in digital health and nursing education and practice. It identified the challenges and benefits of digital health and digital skills as a fundamental pillar of digital health. Digital skills are required to successfully complete your degree and to deliver the best possible care for the patients.

Rapid technological developments and transformation means that the future of all professions, including nursing, will require digital skills. Primary and secondary care settings are integrating more technologies; therefore, the nursing profession must adapt to a future in that caring for the patient is a digitally enabled process. Access to devices, platforms, tools and the data generated through use can enhance nursing practice, facilitate centred care and empower patients to self-manage. It is essential for student nurses to be at the forefront of digital innovation and engage in digital activities and education.

Activities: brief outline answers

Activity 1.3   Advise Yolanda (page 18)

It is important for Yolanda to know her proficiency levels to set up realistic and smart goals specific to areas that she has to improve. She might be more proficient in specific areas (e.g., cybersecurity and online safety) but less proficient with accessing and deciding which sources of information are good for her). In this situation, it is important for Yolanda to focus more on areas specific to information and curation ('Information, data and content', HEE domain).

An example of top tips is outlined below.

1. Use an existing digital tool to self-assess your digital capabilities, identify strengths and opportunities for further personal development.

2. Set up realistic goals for short-, medium- and long-term plan.

3. Identify a course that will help you achieve your goals.

4. Seek other resources and support to help you realise your goal (e.g., a peer, mentor, digital champion, a community of practice).

5. Set up 30 minutes every day to explore a piece of technology, a platform, an app that you are using personally (e.g., mobile banking, social media family group). Consider what transferable skills you already have from day-to-day use of technology.

The future chapters in this book help you to understand more sources of support for Yolanda.

Chapter 2

Digital toolkit: devices, platforms and tools to support your practice

Amanda Miller and Mike Smith

HEE Digital Capabilities Framework

This chapter will address the following domains of digital capability:

Data and content (level 2)

- Use digital tools to search, locate and organise information.

Teaching, learning and self-development (level 2)

- Use digital tools (e.g., devices, digital platforms) for personal learning.

Communication, collaboration (level 2)

- Understand the role of online platforms to communicate, understand different purposes and function of devices and platforms
- Work and collaborate with people digitally using a range of tools and technologies (e.g., document sharing, cloud-storage systems)

Technical proficiency (level 2)

- Use a wide range of technical devices for personal and professional requirements

---

Chapter aims

After reading this chapter, you will be able to:

- identify the various digital devices used in healthcare education and practice;
- recognise the benefits and drawbacks of various digital devices;

- understand the use of wearable devices and extended realities for healthcare;
- identify software, platforms and applications relevant to health education and practice.

Introduction

As a result of the recent advancements in digital technology, being familiar with a variety of digital tools and devices is essential. Nowadays, there are no longer just one or two devices to choose from, and students need to be able to select a device that is suitable for their educational and practice needs. Laptops and desktop computers are still required for many digital tasks, including essay writing, PowerPoint presentations and poster design. However, the continued development and capabilities of smartphones and tablets has meant that students are not always required to carry bulky devices to and from the workplace or university. Furthermore, patient care is evolving rapidly with assessments and treatments regularly conducted using digital or virtual means. It is important that, as healthcare practitioners, you are able to demonstrate technical competence in using a range of devices and digital tools for teaching and learning and clinical practice (HEE, 2018). In this chapter, we will explore the use of different devices, software and platforms, and discuss the associated advantages and disadvantages for students and patients.

Activity 2.1   Reflection

Before we introduce you to the digital tools available, in your own notes write down all the different tools, devices, platforms and applications you use currently for your personal life, your professional life (working or placements) and studying. After you have completed this activity, think about what technology you might be required to use during your nursing programme from a studying and clinical perspective. Some examples are provided in Figure 2.1.

A brief outline answer is provided at the end of this chapter.

Physical devices

Smartphones

Over the last decade, smartphones have evolved as a mobile device used for a variety of purposes, including accessing the internet, filming and photography, secure contactless payments, leisure activities (reading and listening to music), social media and communication. The use of smartphones in higher education is commonplace, with teaching and learning benefits well documented (Crompton and Burke, 2018; Kim et al., 2017). It is almost an expectation that students in higher education have access to a smartphone; O'Connor and Andrews (2018) reported in their study that 98 per cent of students used a smartphone. Further, in nursing undergraduate education, the reported advantages include increased learning satisfaction and an increase in knowledge, skills and confidence in learning (Kim and Park, 2019). Furthermore, in nursing education, the use of the smartphone in the classroom provides students with the ability to access the internet to check understanding and refer to clinical guidelines/policy – for example, the British National Formulary and Lifesaver apps. Specific applications are also aimed at increasing student engagement and interaction, such as Kahoot, Padlet and Mentimeter.

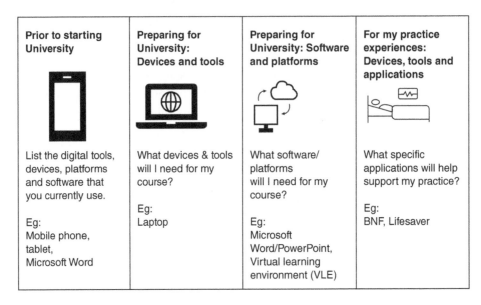

Prior to starting University	Preparing for University: Devices and tools	Preparing for University: Software and platforms	For my practice experiences: Devices, tools and applications
List the digital tools, devices, platforms and software that you currently use. Eg: Mobile phone, tablet, Microsoft Word	What devices & tools will I need for my course? Eg: Laptop	What software/ platforms will I need for my course? Eg: Microsoft Word/PowerPoint, Virtual learning environment (VLE)	What specific applications will help support my practice? Eg: BNF, Lifesaver

Figure 2.1   Examples of digital tools

Smartphone technology is also being used to support students learning in clinical practice, with the reported benefits of having quick access to educational information, reduced anxiety in clinical practice and an improvement in confidence and knowledge (Flynn et al., 2018; O'Connor and Andrews, 2018; Saab et al., 2021). However, some drawbacks of relying on mobile devices in practice include poor Wi-Fi connectivity and a negative attitude towards their use from staff nurses (O'Connor and Andrews, 2018).

In addition, it is important that nursing students have the knowledge and skills relating to smartphone use and be able to provide health and education advice to patients. Over the last two decades Mobile health (m-Health) technology has developed at an exponential rate. The extensive use of personal digital assistants (PDAs), patient monitoring devices and the advanced capabilities of the smartphone has resulted in significant changes in the way that health is assessed, managed and monitored. Further, m-Health has resulted in improved patient–doctor communications, self-management, and the monitoring of disease and better access to healthcare information (Ganasegeran and Abdulrahman, 2019). m-Health applications are considered essential in making healthcare accessible to everyone (WHO, 2011). Examples include the NHS app to access own data, ordering of repeat prescriptions, remote diagnosis, pre-programmed self-assessment health prompts – for example, blood glucose monitoring. Table 2.1 identifies some examples of existing evidence-based applications (apps) aimed at monitoring and promoting health. QR codes have been provided so that you can access the URL of the applications.

Application name	QR code	Purpose	Target audience
Digital Health Passport		Asthma management	Young people with asthma
Hey pharmacist		View, order and manage prescriptions	Adults with regular prescriptions
First Aid by British Red Cross		Provides simple information about first aid	Anyone who wants to learn more about first aid emergencies
MoleCare		Check and monitor moles	Anyone over 4 years old who wants to monitor skin health
My Possible Self: the mental health app		Record and track symptoms related to fear, stress and anxiety	Those over 18 years who experience stress and/or anxiety
mySugr		Track blood sugars, record carbohydrate intake and estimate HbA1c	Those over 16 with diabetes
Hear me now		Helps people with learning disabilities understand information about their health	People with a learning disability

Table 2.1 Example of apps

Case study: Grant

Grant is attending an interactive teaching session on medicines management. One of the exercises involves exploring different types of medications used on a cardiology ward. Using a mobile device, Grant is signposted to several resources to help work through the activities. These include the British National Formulary app and QR codes directly linked to the Professional Guidance on the Administration of Medicines in Healthcare Settings (Royal Pharmaceutical Society, 2019), the Medicines Health Regulatory Authority and the British Pharmaceutical Society.

Activity 2.2   Reflection

Think about the last face-to-face teaching session that you attended. Were you asked to access your phone or tablet during the session? If so, what did you use it for? Was it essential that you had access to a mobile device during the session? Also, consider what else you could have used your phone for during the session. Now make a list of the advantages and disadvantages of mobile phones in the classroom.

A brief outline answer is provided at the end of this chapter.

Tablets

Tablets (or tablet computers) are small, lightweight portable devices that are used generally for browsing the internet, reading books and sending emails. However, certain apps can be installed which increase the ability of the tablet, such as Microsoft Office packages. Tablets generally are touch-screen devices, with built-in features such as camera and GPS. Benefits of tablets are their portability, with no requirement for a keyboard or mouse, good battery life and being relatively more affordable compared to laptops or desktop PCs.

Laptops, desktop computers and storage

Having a laptop or desktop computer is essential for your nursing studies as you will need this for accessing the virtual learning environment (VLE) and producing written work. During your programme, you will be required to complete pieces of formative and summative work, including essays, PowerPoint presentations, poster presentations and reflective written work. Being competent in the use of Microsoft Word and PowerPoint is paramount for your studies. Although such software can be downloaded on to tablets or phones, when writing a long essay or designing a presentation, the use of a laptop or desktop computer enables a larger screen and increased functionality.

Laptop computers are portable, electronic devices that can be used in any environment. The key benefits of using a laptop over a desktop computer is the portability, built-in accessories (keyboard/touchpad mouse/webcam) and many are lightweight and compact. Additional accessories can be purchased for laptops, including external hard drives for increased storage and docking stations. However, laptops have limited storage, a small screen and can be more expensive in comparison to desktop computers, although limited storage can be mitigated through the use of Cloud platforms (for example, OneDrive). Desktop computers are a useful static device with increased power, improved accessibility, larger screens and are cost-effective. There is, however, a shift to move away from using desktop computers in exchange for laptops due to their portability and space-saving capabilities. Figure 2.2 identifies the timeline for the development of computer and smart technology

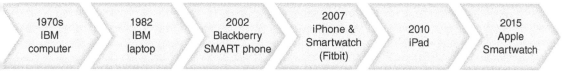

Figure 2.2   Computer and smart technology development timeline

Activity 2.3   Critical thinking

Consider which device or devices would be best for the following scenarios. Provide a rationale for your answers.

Scenario 1

You have been asked to use a new interactive virtual reality platform for one of your practice-based teaching sessions. For this, you are required to download software that requires 8GB RAM and 15GB storage.

Scenario 2

You are currently on placement with the community mental health team. You and your practice assessor are visiting a young person who has recently been discharged following self-harming. You want to point them to some resources that might help support them.

Scenario 3

You are attending a lecture and have been told by the facilitator that there will be some interactive activities, including voting and using a whiteboard. You have been advised to bring an 'electronic device' to the session.

A brief outline answer is provided at the end of this chapter.

Wearables

Over the last decade, smart wearable devices have revolutionised how personal health is measured and monitored. There are various wearable devices that enable monitoring of health behaviour/activity either from a personal or healthcare professional perspective. Such devices include smart watches, smart clothing, head-mounted devices, patches, body sensors and implantable devices (Guk et al., 2019). Rawassizadeh et al. (2015) define the smart watch as a 'general-purpose, networked computer with an array of sensors'. Smart watches can be used for various personal self-management purposes, such as tracking activity/sport, heart rate and sleep/rest cycles. An example of smart watch technology for the healthcare professional includes the ability to alert and monitor falls (Warrington et al., 2021). The advantages of such wearable devices are that they are relatively low cost and accurate for identifying a fall and summoning the appropriate help. Other examples of wearable technology to record health status include:

- patches or watches for blood-pressure monitoring;
- glucose monitoring for those with diabetes;
- balance and tremor monitoring for those with Parkinson's disease;
- wearable clothing to monitor physiological observations.

Wearable devices have the advantage of being able to be monitored remotely by healthcare professionals via telehealth or mobile applications. However, they rely on the individual's commitment to ensure that the device is worn constantly and correctly, and kept charged.

Implantable devices have been in existence since the early 1960s with the first cardiac pacemaker and is the most well-known implantable device. Pacemakers are used to manage and treat arrhythmias. By detecting irregular heartbeats, the pacemaker is able to restore the normal heart rhythm through the delivery of low-energy electrical pulses (Guk et al., 2019). In Parkinson's disease, deep brain stimulators (DBS) are implantable devices that assist with the relief of symptoms including dyskinesia (involuntary movements), tremors and altered gait. A small wire (lead) with four electrodes is implanted in a specific area of the brain responsible for movement. It is connected to a pacemaker inserted into the upper torso and this transmits small electrical currents through the wire regulating the abnormal brain cell activity that causes the symptoms of gait problems and tremor.

Activity 2.4   Reflection

Reflect on your practice experiences. Can you identify other wearable devices that you have seen in use to assist with monitoring and measuring health? What were they used for? Who was the wearable device aimed at?

A brief outline answer is provided at the end of this chapter.

XR and simulation devices

Computerised technology to create simulated environments and scenarios has advanced considerably over the last decade. More specifically, the creation of highly advanced human patient simulators has progressed significantly. In the 1960s, Asmund Laerdal designed one of the first full body simulators – namely, the Resusci Anne – with the ability to practise cardiopulmonary resuscitation skills. Since then, human patient simulators have been developed further to imitate realistic physiological characteristics such as altered chest sounds, heart sounds, palpable pulses and pupillary reactions. Adult, infant, neonatal, child and pregnant models are available, and are used in undergraduate healthcare education. Simulation in nurse education is widely recognised as an effective pedagogy and is described by Gaba (2004):

> *A technique – not a technology – to replace or amplify real experiences with guided experiences that evoke or replicate substantial aspects of the real world in a fully interactive manner.*

Fidelity in simulation refers to the level of realism demonstrated in a simulated practice experience and is described as low-, medium- or high-fidelity simulation. The level of fidelity depends on several components including the environment, the manikin (or simulated patient) and the psychological experience of the learner. An example of low-fidelity simulation is the use of a part-task trainer (a venepuncture arm, catheterisation model) for students to develop their psychomotor skills (Figure 2.3) An example of high-fidelity simulation is the use of a human patient simulator that simulates a complex physiological state (anaphylaxis, asthma or seizures) and responds to treatment initiated by the learner (Figure 2.4).

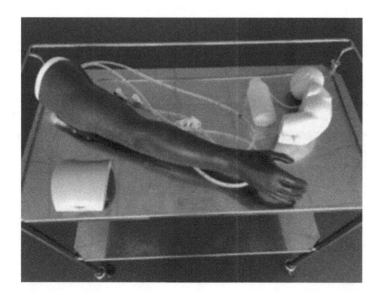

Figure 2.3 A part-task trainer

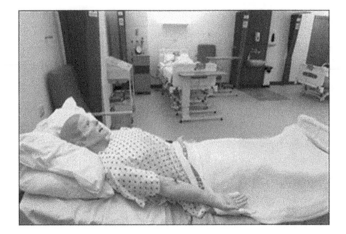

Figure 2.4   Human patient simulator

Higher Education Institutions (HEIs) and Health Education England (HEE) have invested significantly in simulation. The use of this teaching and learning approach is considered integral to nurse education (NMC, 2018b; NMC, 2020). From April 2023, HEE will merge with NHS England, which will strengthen the collaboration between education and practice. The NMC (2018b) identified that simulation can be used proportionately to replace clinical hours. However, following the challenges of the Covid-19 pandemic the NMC stated that HEIs could apply for an amendment to their programmes, allowing a maximum of 600 hours of simulated-based learning to replace direct placement hours (NMC, 2022). More significantly, the definition of simulation-based learning includes virtual and digital experiences, case studies and reflections. This enables HEIs and practice partners much more flexibility and opportunities to deliver innovative and simulated practice experiences.

Extended realities (XR) is a general term used to describe all real and virtual environments created by computer-generated wearables and technology. XR includes virtual reality (VR), augmented reality (AR) and mixed reality (MR). Virtual reality enables the learner to be immersed in an artificial 3D or 2D world. This is most commonly experienced through the use of VR headsets – for example, Oculus – or immersive projected environments (Figure 2.5).

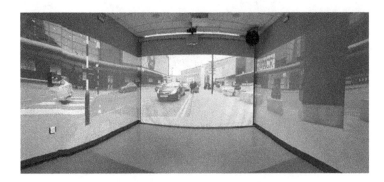

Figure 2.5   Immersive projected environments

Software and platforms

Generic software

While the devices we use and their functionality is important, what really makes them useful is the software we use on them and how we can get the best out of this. There are some generic programs that you already likely use every day that often aren't being used to their full potential. When working at their best, software and our devices should help us with our lives, not add an extra burden to our work. Often, this comes down to how we are using them and whether we are using all the features effectively and the right program for the job we are doing.

Let's start by looking at one of the most commonly used types of software, which are word processors. You will more commonly know these as Microsoft Word or Google Documents, but many others are available. If you are someone who is not particularly a quick typist or perhaps you have problems with spelling because of learning needs like dyslexia, using dictation or speech to text functions can be really helpful. Within Microsoft 365 you can find the dictate function on the home taskbar or in Google Documents you can find this in tools and voice typing. These can be incredibly useful functions as well if you articulate yourself better at talking rather than typing. It can depend on how well the software can recognise your voice and accurately record the words you are saying.

The reverse of this can also be useful as software packages have text-to-speech functions, which means that the computer will read your text aloud to you. Where this is particularly useful is when you come to proofread your work and spot mistakes. Often we don't recognise mistakes when looking at them on-screen, but having the computer read aloud the words that you've actually typed rather than the words you believe you have typed can be a very effective way to identify these mistakes.

When we write longer documents such as reports or dissertations, managing how this is broken down is important. Rather than just underlining headings or subheadings, we can use the automated styles for the titles and subheadings. This has the benefit of ensuring that your document has consistency in that style, as well as when it comes to creating your table of contents. This can be as simple as clicking on the Table of Contents function (in Microsoft Word you will find this under the References tab, in Google Documents you will find this under the Insert menu).

Activity 2.5 Reflection

Experiment with these features for whichever word-processing software you are using. You can also try to see how long it takes you to type out a particular section of text compared

(Continued)

(Continued)

to how long it takes you to dictate it. You may find this is a more useful way for you to go about constructing your assignments.

A brief outline answer is provided at the end of this chapter.

Cloud solutions

Increasingly, the usefulness of our physical devices is not necessarily what is on them or what they do, but their ability to connect to the internet and other devices. Traditionally, we would save our files to our own devices and, when needed, we would store them on portable media like USB drives. This is largely being replaced with what is known as Cloud Storage. What this term means is that instead of being on one device, it is saved to the internet across one or more large data centres. The benefit of this is that it can be accessed at any time from any device, provided you have access to the internet. This is an excellent way to store important files such as essays or documents you do not want to lose, as even if your computer breaks or is lost, you can still access the files from anywhere. Documents stored online typically have autosave enabled on them so any changes you make are automatically updated, which removes the problem of having forgotten to save your work.

Activity 2.6a   Communication

Save or create a new document in a Cloud Storage area. You will likely already have one set up with your university, but if not Microsoft OneDrive and Google Drive offer free versions of this. Ensure that you know how to access this on different devices.

https://onedrive.live.com/about/en-gb/signinR
https://drive.google.com/drive/my-drive

A brief outline answer is provided at the end of this chapter.

One of the most common Cloud Storage platforms you will come across as a student is the university virtual learning environment. Some common examples of this are Blackboard or Moodle. As a minimum, these act as a central point for all the learning materials you will engage with on your course. These platforms may also be how you will access live online sessions, discussion boards and asynchronous material such as recorded presentations. It is useful to become familiar with these and the layout your organisation uses so you can locate the resources easily. As most readers will be aware, one of the outcomes that came from the Covid-19 lockdown was the more widespread adoption of online learning. While it was recognised that some elements of this were not as effective, sessions that are aimed purely at providing information such as lectures have been found to be better delivered as a recorded online learning session, as they provide a number of benefits, including captions (subtitles), flexibility of when you access them and the ability to rewatch sections or the whole session as you wish.

Often, we equate learning to the time we spend in a classroom with a teacher talking to, or in the worst case, at us. This didactic approach to teaching is increasingly recognised as not the best way for people to learn. Especially within nursing, we want students to learn the skills to think critically for themselves and to work collaboratively in teams. Collaborative learning is a recognised and valuable way to work with others to learn together (Zhang and Cui, 2018). With the growth in blended approaches to learning in universities and collaboration on work in healthcare, the ability to share the work we are doing in real time is becoming an expectation rather than an optional extra. Rather than working against collaborative approaches, technology can be used to supplement and enhance that collaboration. This might be in the form of virtual meetings, which can be especially useful when students do not live in the same geographical area, as well as shared documents that can be used when students are separate or when students are together working on the same document. Some examples of these shared documents might be group projects or shared note-taking from classes.

Activity 2.6b   Communication

Set up a document on your Cloud Storage with nursing terminology and explanations you have come across. Share this with some of your peers. This is usually done by opening the share options in the software where you can select if you want people to be able to view the file or be able to edit it; you will need others to be able to edit this document. You will then have the option of sending the invitation to others either by copying a link or sending them access directly via their email.

As you all find new terminology, you can share and add to this document. As well as benefitting from sharing what each of you has found out, this can be a way for people to share what they know and where one person might post a new term that they are unfamiliar with, another can add detail as to what it means, as well as posting links to further information.

A brief outline answer is provided at the end of this chapter.

Social media platforms

The final area of Cloud Storage which we will touch on in this chapter is that of social media. If it were not already apparent how integrated Cloud computing is with our lives, then social media is likely to be the most obvious example. Being as hyper-connected as we all are has both advantages and disadvantages, which we will explore in more detail as we go through the other chapters. Some of the negative effects of this are that some nurses have broken confidentiality or presented unprofessional behaviour or opinions, which has led to questions about their suitability for their role. Some positive examples of how we might interact with these as nurses are networking opportunities, access to information we wouldn't be able to gain otherwise, as well as other opportunities for research or developing services.

For patients, there are some potential negative effects, such as social media exposing people to bullying and misinformation (Gabbaron et al., 2021; O'Reilly, 2020) as well as a potentially overwhelming amount of information, particularly for patients who are newly diagnosed. However, it can confer a host of benefits, including allowing them to connect to people who may be experiencing similar conditions to them and access support for managing their health (Simms, 2020). The anonymity allowed by some social media allows people to feel more comfortable in accessing information and seeking support around stigmatised conditions such as mental health issues (O'Reilly et al., 2019). The ability to engage with peer support allows people not to feel alone with their condition, access the types of advice that comes from the lived experience of having the condition, as well as better understanding of their condition. This leaves people better equipped and more confident in managing their own health (Vasilica et al., 2020).

Activity 2.7   Reflection

While social media is not preferred by all people, it can be helpful for patients and clinicians. Please visit the following sites:

> **https://kinet.site/blogs**
> **www.facebook.com/DementiaFriends**
> **www.tiktok.com/@dr.karanr**

Reflect on the following questions:

1. Should social media be used by patients to share their lived experiences?
2. Are social media platforms (e.g., TikTok or YouTube) useful platforms to disseminate public health information?
3. Reflect on your own social media presence. Does it reflect that of a professional person?

A brief outline answer is provided at the end of this chapter.

XR and simulation software packages

There are specific XR programs that have been created for nursing and healthcare education – for example, Second Life®, Body Interact® and Oxford Medical Simulation® (OMS). OMS is designed to be used with a headset or standard computers. Learners are able to interact with virtual acutely unwell patients and are expected to assess and manage their care within an episode of care. Once learners have completed the scenario, they can receive feedback, performance metrics and participate in a reflective guided debrief. VR headsets enable the student to be immersed into a simulated environment and experience a 360-degree first-person perspective. However, the drawbacks of the VR headset is affordability and accessibility. Alternative, less costly cardboard headset options are available and work in conjunction with smartphones. While VR uses 3D technology to mimic the real world, augmented reality is a technology that superimposes digital information such as sounds, images or text over a real setting to enhance the sensory experience.

Internet search and organising

While you are studying, there are numerous pieces of software and web-based services aimed at supporting students and academic work. One that we urge students to get to grips with early are journal databases. These initially work like a normal search engine in that you initially enter keywords into the search bar and it retrieves results for you. Where this differs is that because it is a curated database, you can be assured that the sources are of high academic quality and so you can use them as evidence for your practice as a nurse and also for academic work.

Unlike most search engines, you can also use the other features to make your life much easier by filtering out the articles you aren't interested in. Most commonly, you would only want to retrieve articles in the last ten years, so you are using contemporary sources. You may also want to select only articles that are written in English or those that have a full text available.

Some other tips are:

- Be aware of different spellings of the same word such as 'behaviour' and 'behavior'.
- Use the Boolean operators features of AND, OR and NOT, which are sometimes found in the advanced search options. These allow you to look at the specific topic you are researching. For example, if you were looking at wound care for people with diabetes, but weren't focusing on complications from infections, you would search for 'Diabetes' AND 'Wound care' NOT infections.
- Use the filters to further get rid of results that you aren't interested in. Some commonly used filters are: date published (usually we would only use work published in the last ten years), full paper texts available, language it is written in, country of origin.

Activity 2.8   Reflection

Locate one of your university's nursing databases. Some examples of these are CINAHL and Medline. How you navigate to these will depend on the university. If you are unsure, please make enquiries with your tutor or the library. Use the suggestions above to help you locate a journal article on a subject you are interested in.

A brief outline answer is provided at the end of this chapter.

When you are studying, you will often find that it is difficult to keep track of the references you have used. To help with this, there are many reference management services and systems available such as RefWorks, EndNote and EasyBib. These can help to generate the reference for you and can store your reference list to be exported directly into your work as well. Some things to be cautious of are to ensure that the software is set to the style of referencing that your university or school uses. There are many different styles, so it is worth double-checking. In addition to this, the reference that it will generate can occasionally have errors, so you still need to know how to reference accurately yourself in order to check it.

Healthcare systems

As well as the more generic pieces of software, there is specific software that is useful in practice for both staff and patients in the form of electronic health records, which are systems that store information about the care received by individuals accessing NHS services (Jacob, 2020). There are numerous benefits of having electronic record systems as opposed to paper-based systems. For staff, these can range from being able to access the same records at the same time as staff in other areas, allowing for easier communication or looking back at historic information without the delays of having to locate the previous paper-based notes. What this means for patient care is that decisions are not delayed by not having access to notes or that relevant information is not missing which could be vitally important to decision making, as is illustrated in the case of Travis below.

Case study: Travis

Laura is a community nurse who has been asked to see a new patient, Travis, whom she has not met before. Laura is able to use her work computer from her car to see that Travis has recently been discharged from the hospital and can look back at all other relevant history as well as information about how to access Travis's house. When Laura goes to see Travis, she finds him to be extremely unwell and recognises that he is showing signs of sepsis. Once Travis is sent to the hospital, she is able to record her observations in his notes. Travis is taken to a different hospital than he was previously admitted. However, staff there are able to see what the community nurse has observed, what has recently happened, as well as importantly that he is severely allergic to the antibiotic they would have prescribed to him.

Chapter summary

In summary, we have briefly explored ways in which different aspects of technology will play a part in the role of the nurse and how they can be beneficial to the role and to yourself as a student. There is no doubt that the use of digital tools in healthcare will continue to grow as time goes on. While there are clear benefits to this hyper-connected world we live in, we have to have the skills to take advantage of them fully and also to avoid the risks that can come with them. Throughout the subsequent chapters, we will explore how you can go about this. One of the messages we would like people to take away from this chapter is that these devices and services are there as tools for you to use, as, just like any other tool practice, it means that you can get the best from them. When there is a new system or device that you come across in practice or your day-to-day life, explore its features to see what it can do and how you can use this to support what you do. Don't limit yourself to just knowing how to do the bare minimum. Find out why you have to do something in a certain way, be curious and embrace them as tools to help rather than see them as hoops to jump through.

Activities: brief outline answers

For the reflective activities, there are no correct or incorrect answers, but below are some of the expected themes that might have been raised by these activities.

Activity 2.1   Reflection (page 21)

Your personal use will be particular to you. Within nursing, we use electronic record systems that include written notes as well as visual data like X-rays, electronic observation machines and video calling as a few examples.

Activity 2.2   Reflection (page 24)

Advantages are: access to wider research, interaction to ask questions or answer questions (e.g., quizzes), encouraging students to be curious about what they are discussing. Disadvantages are: distractions looking at things rather than paying attention to what is happening in the session, interruptions from messages and phone calls, barriers to in-person communication.

Activity 2.3   Reflection (page 25)

Scenario 1: A laptop or VR headset depending on the nature of the platform. It may be that the requirements of the software may be more than some lower-end tablets.

Scenario 2: Tablet or mobile phone as internet access will likely be needed in places where you may not have access to Wi-FI. Tablets have the benefit that they are easier to see with bigger screens.

Scenario 3: Laptop, tablet or mobile phone. They are all compatible, but may be easier to view and interact on larger devices.

Activity 2.4   Reflection (page 26)

Example: Step counter/activity tracker – generally aimed at fit and healthy people or able-bodied people seeking to be more active.

Activity 2.5   Reflection (page 29)

See which way works best for you. It can be a matter of personal preference about what works best for you or for particular situations.

Activity 2.6a and 2.6b   Reflection (pages 30 and 31)

Try this and note how it makes collaboration easier, particularly when studying from home so you don't have to be on campus to stay connected with your peers.

Activity 2.7   Reflection (page 32)

1. It can help people not to feel alone with their conditions. However, people tend to share the times when it isn't going well, so this can be detrimental.

2. Yes, but can also be shown alongside misinformation that can be confusing and doesn't get people to think about the quality of the source they get information from.

3. If a patient were to look back at your profile, would they think you were a safe and responsible person?

Activity 2.8   Reflection (page 34)

Using these systems and features can make your studying much easier. However, you do need to get familiar with them to get the benefit.

Chapter 3 · Looking after the digital well-being of yourself and others

Nicky Varley and Kirstie Harrison

HEE Digital Capabilities Framework

This chapter will address the following domains of digital capability:

Digital identity, well-being, safety and security (level 2)

- Develop, promote and safeguard appropriate digital identity(-ies) that support a positive personal and organisational reputation
- Use digital technologies in ways that support personal well-being and safety and the well-being and safety of others
- Recognise and act upon digital situations and events that might compromise personal, professional or organisational security

Teaching, learning and self-development (level 2)

- Use a range of digital tools and technologies in my online learning – e.g., podcasts, video tutorials, online courses
- Review personal learning and identify new areas for development

Communication, collaboration and participation (level 2)

- Follow guidance and regulations that apply to appropriate online/digital communication and participation.

Chapter aims

After reading this chapter, you will be able to:

- reflect on your personal and professional use of digital technologies;
- identify changes you can make to enhance your own digital well-being;
- understand your role as a professional nurse in looking after the digital well-being of others;
- recognise negative situations involving digital technologies and take action in alignment with your professional responsibilities as a nurse.

Introduction

In this hyperconnected world, digital well-being remains a priority, whether that is related to using digital devices to improve well-being or maintaining a healthy relationship with technology. In this chapter, those two aspects of digital well-being are explored. As health professionals, it is important to understand the utility of technology to improve outcomes for patients and the public, including safe use of the internet, protection against cyberbullying, misused information and cybersecurity.

Similarly, these concepts are important at a personal level to safely participate in online communities and networks, act in accordance with the nursing code of practice, establish norms and negotiate conflict, manage digital workload and overall be in a safe online space. Personal growth can emerge from choosing to take control of your own digital well-being and by supporting the digital well-being of others.

Digital well-being

What is the first thing that comes into your mind when you hear the term 'digital well-being'? For some, it might be countless emails containing offers that just cannot be missed, fake news or Instagram ads. Perhaps it is your fitness tracker that reminds you how many steps you have left to reach your daily goal or analyses if you are getting quality sleep.

The *Oxford Dictionary* (2021) defines well-being as *the state of being comfortable, healthy and happy* and defines wellness as the *state of being in good health, especially as an actively pursued goal.*

Consider the role that technologies and digital activities play in your daily life and the term 'digital well-being' will now feel far more relevant to you. It is important to consider the impact that these have on physical, mental, social and emotional well-being and how far these might affect an individual and those around you in a personal and professional context.

According to JISC (2019), it is widely agreed that digital well-being is a multifaceted concept with various perspectives to consider.

Individual

This refers to your own personal work–life balance. It is important that you are involved in identifying the positive benefits and understanding any potential detrimental aspects that may arise when you are involved in digital activities, and how to manage your own health and well-being when accessing and utilising digital technology.

Societal/organisational

Organisations that are providing digital systems and services have a duty to ensure that these digital applications are well managed and accessible. Furthermore, organisations must be able to empower and support users who engage with their technology to support the individual's health and well-being.

Activity 3.1   Reflection

Thinking about the above perspectives, begin to reflect on your own digital well-being as an individual. It is possible that you may never have taken time to reflect on this concept. Now think about how your digital well-being might compare to that of your patients and that of the organisation you work for. Do we take the time to consider this perspective when we care for ourselves and others?

An outline answer is provided at the end of this chapter.

Your digital presence

Central to nursing is patient advocacy and protecting your patients from harm. This includes their digital well-being. Public health is an integral part of nursing education and practice and as student nurses/nurses, we must safeguard patient information whether written, verbal or digital.

Once you enter the profession as a student, you sign up to a way of life, to promote health and prevent ill-health, improve safety and quality and, above all, be an accountable professional (Nursing and Midwifery Council [NMC], 2018a). There are other platforms to consider here, but the three listed are particularly linked to the importance of the digital well-being of others.

As healthcare environments are progressively becoming embedded with digital technology, there is now a focus on healthcare professionals developing their digital professionalism which will form part of their professional identity. While there is currently no standard definition of the term, digital professionalism has become a familiar term in response to the need for healthcare professionals to increase their awareness and develop their understanding of the appropriate professional behaviour standards when using digital platforms.

The term 'digital footprint' is used to describe everything you do online, from using social media platforms such as Twitter, Instagram and Facebook to submitting your assignments through your university portal. Every click, share, photo, tweet and 'like' are permanent indentations on your digital footprint. As a student nurse/nurse or health professional, being vigilant is imperative to you and the profession you are registered to.

Scenario A

You are sitting in a local café near to the hospital where you and your peers are on placement. One of them starts to discuss a patient they were working with that day. Your peer tells you and the others that he had been reading the patient notes, then proceeds to discuss the patient by name and discloses personal information about where they live, their history and the patient's family.

Scenario B

You follow a TikTok account which follows the journey of a student nurse. You see a video talking about an experience with a patient. The user mentions the first name of the patient and does an impression of them. There are a variety of positive and negative comments on the video, including one from an identifiable qualified nurse who says, 'Ha-ha, I know XX only too well. This impression of one of her tantrums is perfect!'

Activity 3.2   Patient confidentiality and respect

Reading the scenarios above:

- What are things to consider here?
- How would you handle each situation?
- Would you have a different response in this digital scenario (B) compared to the in-person scenario (A)?

An outline answer is provided at the end of this chapter.

Professional vs. personal dentity

A digital identity is a body of information regarding an individual or an organisation that exists online. Your digital identity is created organically from the personal information on the internet and the data accessed by an individual online (Guraya et al., 2021).

Have you ever searched for a person on the web? Your friend, your partner, yourself or even your new boss? You can easily do this online, but remember the same can easily be done by your manager and even the patients and their families that we care for. Therefore, the way you present yourself to the digital community must be considered with the knowledge that your present and past online behaviour may be accessed by a variety of individuals.

The Nursing and Midwifery Social Media Guidance (2019), which is underpinned by the NMC *Code* (2018a) is a useful starting point that encourages students and qualified staff to read in conjunction with their employers' social media policy. While the guidance issued by the NMC acknowledges that social media is constantly evolving and while it is not intended to cover every social media scenario you may face, it does set out the broad principles that will encourage and assist you in thinking about your own digital identity, issues you may face and the importance of acting professionally at all times to ensure the public's protection at all times.

Activity 3.3   Understanding your digital footprint

Have you ever googled yourself? Try it and see what type of information you are sharing via your online platforms and what can be accessed openly. It's worth trying this on a device you do not use often – for example, a library computer, as this will show a more realistic view of what others might see if they searched for you. Are you sending the correct message to the online community about yourself? In what ways would you like to see your digital footprint change?

An outline answer is provided at the end of this chapter.

Social media is a useful tool when thinking about your professional identity: it is a way of expressing your character and personality, an alternative portal for others to get a sense of your character and personality. It is also a way to build interpersonal relationships and create or strengthen professional networks (Gabbard, 2019). Therefore, having a well-controlled online presence will allow you to showcase your abilities and your professional interests. Many people do hold a personal and professional social media account. However, you need to be aware that while your professional account is readily viewable by the public, there is still a chance that the online community may find and view your personal accounts. Therefore, it is important to ensure that you safeguard these personal accounts too. While nobody is telling you that you cannot have fun away from work, you are responsible for preventing yourself and your profession from falling into disrepute by your behaviour.

Top tips for health professionals to stay safe online

1. Manage who can see you on social media.

2. Think before you post or tweet as a rule of thumb. Think, is it truthful, kind, necessary?

3. Don't vent your anger on social media.

4. Don't discuss patients, where you work or people you work with on social media.

5. Remember, if you are in a social media 'group', they are still an audience.

6. Don't give out any personal information.

7. Pick safe and secure passwords.

Lastly, if used correctly, social media is great for networking. Try searching for #WeStNs or #WeNurses on Twitter or explore the we communities website for other useful networks.

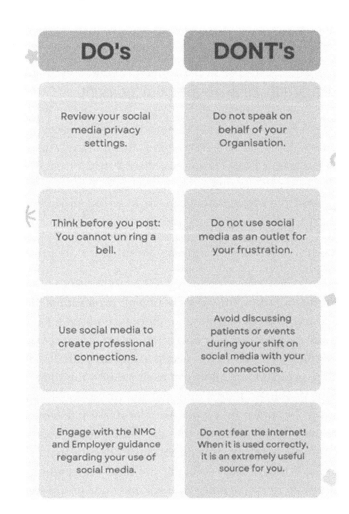

Figure 3.1   Do's and don'ts of staying safe online

Nurse–patient relationship

Did you know that users of health services are now, more than ever, turning to the digital space to explore their encounters of care (NHS Digital, 2022)?

As a student or a Registered Nurse, it is important to recognise that the responsibility to maintain boundaries remains with you, as the professional, and not the patient. While engaging in conversations is useful when sharing best practice or perhaps the latest research on a topic, you should be aware of the difference between a dialogue that occurs between two healthcare professionals and a chat between a patient and yourself. With or without social media, the concept of professional boundaries remains the same. A professional boundary is defined as the space between the nurses' power and the patient's vulnerability (Day-Calder, 2019). It may be useful to think about power in terms of 'old' and 'new' within your organisation here. Bailey and Burhouse (2019) discuss how old power can be seen as hierarchical and transactional; people are held to account in a rational way for quality improvement, standards, policies and performance agreements. Therefore, in terms of old power, it could be argued that you have the power within the nurse–patient relationship and therefore it is your responsibility to establish and maintain these boundaries. However, now consider the following in terms of 'new' power: new power motivates people to participate through aligning with their morals and values, and giving them the energy and platform to create change. New power is peer-driven and participatory rather than hierarchical and transactional. Under this new power, 'super connectors' are born. According to Bailey and Burhouse (2019), super connectors:

- will have the relationships, networks, content and context;
- will drive the perceptions of other people;
- are the go-to people for advice;
- make sense of things and reduce ambiguity for others;
- are trusted by peers more than formal leaders are trusted;
- are largely unknown to formal leaders.

Now think about the above qualities and ask yourself: why is it important to ensure that I create and manage professional boundaries within the nurse–patient relationship? In order to identify and build a shared purpose, this is not just about holding the power in a relationship; it is about identifying why there needs to be a boundary set, the positive impact this has on your patient and yourself, and, while there are factors that unite you both in this relationship, the purpose of this relationship is ultimately to help the patient achieve their own state of wellness which is individual to them, while you are able to ensure that you protect your own digital well-being. Read the case study below and consider how this may influence your own nursing practice in the future.

Case study: Emma

Emma is a registered nurse working in a chemotherapy suite. Her patient, Susan, has regularly attended chemotherapy once a week for a course of six weekly cycles. During this time, Emma is able to develop a therapeutic relationship with Susan. They discuss Susan's fears and worries about the treatment, while Emma listens empathetically, offering her advice based on her own experiences caring for individuals who are similar to Susan. Susan asks Emma about her life and Emma is happy to disclose that she has two children of primary school age and lives with her husband and their pet dog. After Susan's chemotherapy cycle is over, Emma wishes her well and all the best at her next consultant meeting.

Later that week, Emma receives a Facebook friend request from Susan: Emma is unsure whether to accept this or not.

Activity 3.4   Reflection

Reflect on the case study and note down your thoughts on the following questions:

1. What is Emma's intent when accepting this friend's request and creating this connection?
2. Is accepting the request in Susan's best interests?
3. Is there a better alternative?

An outline answer is provided at the end of this chapter.

Cyberbullying

What is cyberbullying? In short, it is bullying that is conducted via a digital device. This could be a mobile phone, computer or tablet via any online forum, including text messages, apps, gaming and social media platforms. What might cyberbullying look like? This could be posting, sharing or inciting harmful, false or negative/derogatory content about another person, including sharing personal or private information. In some instances, cyberbullying can be investigated if the behaviour has become unlawful or even criminal in nature. It is important as professionals that we are aware of this. It is built into the NMC *Code of Conduct* (2018a) which states: *the nursing workforce should be treated with dignity, respect and enabled to raise concerns without fear of detriment, and to have these concerns responded to.*

Bullying of any description should never be condoned. If, as professionals, we come across bullying or we are told about bullying, it is important that we act responsibly and seek further help.

Where might cyberbullying take place:

- Social Media, such as Facebook, Instagram, Snapchat, and Tik Tok.
- Text messaging and messaging apps on mobile or tablet devices.
- Instant messaging, direct messaging and online chatting over the internet.
- Online forums, chat rooms and message boards.
- Email.
- Online gaming communities.

Case study: Stacey

Stacey is a third-year student nurse who is currently on placement within an endoscopy clinic. During her third week, Rachel, a second-year student nurse from the same university joins them for a spoke day on the unit. The sister asks Stacey to work with Rachel as they follow a patient journey through endoscopy.

The following day, Stacey is sent a screenshot of a Facebook status by Rachel which reads:

> *Working alongside a third-year student nurse yesterday. The amount of stupid questions she asks and the time it takes for her to complete nursing documentation is beyond a joke!*

Stacey is extremely upset about this comment and contacts a tutor at university who immediately reassures her that she has acted in the correct way escalating this, requests that the screenshot is forwarded to the tutor in order for a fitness to practise referral to be initiated.

Activity 3.5   Reflection

Reflect on the case study above. What do you understand by the term 'fitness to practise' (FtP)? Take some time to locate your university's FtP policy and read through the document. This will help you understand what constitutes an FtP and the process that your university will follow.

An outline answer is provided at the end of this chapter.

Make every contact count

How can we protect our patients from cyberbullying? As nurses and student nurses, every encounter with a patient, group of people or community counts.

It is rare that a patient will present to healthcare professionals with a complaint of bullying, so it is essential that as healthcare professionals, we are aware of the common signs and symptoms that are associated with bullying. These signs and symptoms can include, but are not limited, to the following:

- avoiding school or employment;
- increased anxiety, lower self-esteem;
- reports of sudden withdrawal at home;
- unusual behaviour – e.g., rage or anger;
- self-destructive behaviour;
- reporting health problems – e.g., headaches, abdominal pain.

As you may be aware, *Making Every Contact Count* [MECC] (NHS Education England, 2016), is an approach that uses the millions of day-to-day interactions that occur between healthcare professionals and service users to support them in making positive changes to their physical and mental health and well-being. An MECC interaction takes minutes and is aimed to provide a structured approach to maximise the opportunity within routine health and care interaction to allow your patient to discuss any health or well-being factors that are taking place.

It is widely acknowledged that psychosocial factors and an individual's mental health problem can directly impact on the individual's physical health outcomes.

As a student or a nurse, take time during a appointment or an admission to screen for these signs and symptoms: Vaillancourt et al. (2016) suggest that it may be better to ask a service user about their exposure to cyberbullying using a questionnaire approach rather than asking them directly. It is important to note that victims of cyberbullying are also bullied in traditional ways, and therefore screening for both types of experiences should be considered by the healthcare professional. Research conducted by Ramney et al. (2016) found that screening for cyberbullying can be undertaken in a variety of clinical settings and should not be simply saved, for example, with an acute presentation to the Emergency Department and that school-based, home environments, clinics and inpatient hospital stays are appropriate settings to address bullying.

Activity 3.6   Reviewing clinical practice guidance

Review the screening/admissions/care plans you have accessed in clinical practice. Do they provide guidance on approaching the topic of cyberbullying with a patient? How would you feel addressing this topic with a patient who presented with anxiety and reported headaches?

An outline answer is provided at the end of this chapter.

How cyber safe are you?

Cyber security is the means by which individuals and organisations reduce the risk of being affected by cybercrime (National Cyber Security Agency, 2020).

The essence of cyber security is to safeguard the devices we use daily and the services that are accessible online, both at work and from home. As part of modern life, it is difficult to imagine how we would function without a smart device, the internet or a computer, and therefore it is necessary that we take steps that prevent cyber criminals accessing our accounts, data and devices.

The NHS is made up of more than 8,000 organisations with many more across the wider health and care sector. This makes maintaining robust cyber security a challenge. According to Williams et al. (2019), the risk of a cyber breach reflects factors such as limited resources and fragmented governance. For example, many NHS Trusts spend approximately 1–2 per cent of their annual budget on IT, compared with other sectors whose spend is 4–10 per cent. Reflective of this low-level investment, there are NHS organisations still utilising Windows XP, a Microsoft-operative system that Microsoft ceased to support in 2014. However, the NHS Digital Data Security and Protection Toolkit has been developed to support organisations in identifying vulnerabilities and implementing plans to overcome any identified areas of high risk. These assessments allow the organisation to not only improve their cyber security, but also achieve Cyber Essentials Plus Accreditation while also preparing for the cyber security element of the CQC inspection.

How much is too much?

Research conducted by Lachman (2013) found that many nurses are ignorant of the privacy settings of their social media accounts and are unaware of the distance that their posts on social media can reach. If we do not employ the correct privacy settings on our social media accounts, there is a realm of information that is available to an individual who simply searches your name. This information may include your personal contact information, your religious or political affiliation, relationship status, your health issues, lifestyle choices and even your own personal photographs. It is important to stress that sometimes privacy settings can create a false sense of security: once you press 'send' on that post and it has been published online, sometimes even the most strict settings cannot prevent your post from being shared or duplicated.

Technostress

It is widely recognised that the workload for healthcare professionals is high. Research by Kremer et al. (2019) acknowledged that nurses and medics are reporting high stress levels due to their working environment, placing demands on the individuals to perform a variety of tasks simultaneously. Nurses are reporting higher levels of work-related stress that can create negative physical and psychological effects for themselves as well as their patients (Keykaleh et al., 2018).

First defined in 1984, the term 'technostress' is defined as a modern disease caused by the inability to cope with new computer technologies in a healthy manner (Brod, 1984). Technostress occurs when people are subjected to information overload and

Assemble your
Cyber Secure Tool Box

Limit what you share

Be mindful about the amount of personal information you share online. Review your social media: Your birthday, mobile number, address: Do they appear online?

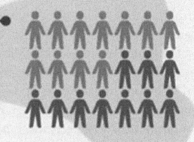

Check! Check again!

How often do you check your account and financial statements? Try to do this on a regular basis. Signing up to a free credit report can also help.

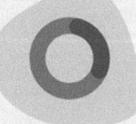

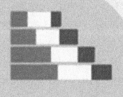

Antivirus, malware and firewalls

Antivirus software is important to protect your device such as computers, laptops or mobiles from malicious softwares that can corrupt your files and data.

Password Manager

How safe is your password? Using a password manager, upper and lower letter, numbers and special characteristics, as well as, two - factor authentification can strengthen your privacy settings

Figure 3.2 Assembling your cyber secure toolbox

repeated contact with digital devices that creates an abnormal response characterised by specific symptoms at cardiovascular, mental and neurological levels. For example, multitasking can lead to hyperarousal of the body's biochemical compositions which can dull the senses. By increasing an individual's stress levels, it can decrease one's sense of control, proving it difficult to think clearly, thus reducing productivity.

Activity 3.7 Reflection

Take your time here to reflect on a typical shift. What does this look like in terms of your use of technology? How many different digital technologies do you utilise in caring for your patients?

As this activity is based on your own reflection no answer is given at the end of this chapter.

During a typical shift, you may find that you are updating your nursing risk assessments, documentations and handovers electronically, monitor and update a patient's observations with technology, triage, send an email, telephone or video consultations, online referral pathways, the work within a virtual ward, access a Trust policy, double-check the dosage of a medication online, log in to your Practice Assessment Documentation, undertake medication rounds, locate a patient's previous hospital notes, set up intravenous fluids through a device, log in to your e-learning, access your rota and keep your mandatory training up to date. The use of information technology has now become complex, pervasive and requires the nurse to be able to process information simultaneously, utilising different devices and technology when providing patient care. Research conducted by Monterio et al. (2017) found that the multiple tasks that nursing staff are required to undertake are frequently interrupted, and dealing with malfunctioning devices coupled with the information overload can lead to the individual becoming overwhelmed, confused and frustrated.

Do you have a healthy digital diet?

When considering your own health and well-being, the amount of time you spend on social media, doing assignments, reading documents or browsing is important. Depending on how you work will depend on whether you spend long periods of time attached to a screen, it is important to take a break. Call a friend, go for a walk, make a drink or just get up and walk away. Your work will still be there in fifteen minutes' time; you will be more productive for it and feel refreshed and ready to start again. One analogy that you may be familiar with is the aeroplane and the oxygen mask: at times of low pressure, you will be instructed to fit your own mask before assisting others with theirs. In life, we all have our own oxygen mask which makes up our energy, time and resources. If we prioritise ourselves first, then we will have more of these resources in reserve to help other people. Similarly, if you don't look after yourself, you may find that you experience overload and this can lead to emotional stress and negatively affect your mental health. It is fine to burn the candle at both ends occasionally, but if this becomes regular practice, you could be heading for 'burnout', so consider putting time aside to do something to boost your well-being. A study conducted by Andrews et al. (2020) found that nurses who proactively engaged with self-care and self-compassion activities were able to manage their emotions effectively while facilitating patients' needs. Results of this study also showed that those nurses who prioritise self-care could prevent negative consequences of nursing, such as burnout and compassion fatigue.

Using social media as a student nurse/nurse, as you have already read in this chapter, can have huge benefits to you both personally and at an organisational level, but it is important to consider that your digital footprint – the video, image or comment on Twitter that you made – is there for everyone to see, so you should respect your profession, and protect yourself and your registration (NMC, 2018a).

It is not surprising that the sophistication of software and the ever-increasing availability of information means that many of us are spending hours in front of a screen each day. Now add this to the time we will spend looking at our own devices and it could be argued we spend the majority of our waking day staring at pixels.

Activity 3.8   Analyse your digital diet

Take a moment for yourself to reflect on your current relationship with technology. Review the statements below and consider if you rarely, sometimes, or often agree:

Statement	Tick which applies to you		
I tend to lose track of time when I am online.	Rarely	Sometimes	Often
If my phone rings, I must check it immediately.	Rarely	Sometimes	Often
When I am with family, I am distracted as I am online.	Rarely	Sometimes	Often
I spend more time online than I would like to.	Rarely	Sometimes	Often
I plan on going to sleep but I stay on my phone instead.	Rarely	Sometimes	Often
I feel like I am missing out if I do not check my social media regularly.	Rarely	Sometimes	Often
If I am asked a question and I do not know the answer, I automatically reach for my phone.	Rarely	Sometimes	Often

(Google, 2020)

Examine your thoughts and feelings now that you have completed this self-assessment. How many times have you ticked 'Often'? Take a moment to reflect on your answers and then

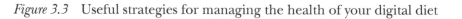

Useful strategies to increase the health of your digital diet

Tap to Shhh. With one tap on your phone, Do Not Disturb will hide all notifications so you won't see them on screen.

1

Shhh

Set a limit! If you want to limit the amount of time you spend on certain websites or apps, why don't you set a daily timer? When the timer runs out, the app is paused for the rest of the day.

2

Have a snooze The snooze function on your smart phone allows you to temporarily hide notifications to give you that short break you might just need.

3

zzZ

Remind yourself Setting your own reminders as often as you need to pause what you are currently accessing on the internet to encourage you to step away regularly.

4

Log off from work By logging out of work profiles and accounts when you finish work, may help you find that balance you could be looking for. Some devices will allow you to schedule them in advance to turn on and off automatically.

5

Finally... Do it together!

It's easier to commit to digital downtime if you make an agreement with friends, family or colleagues. Plus it benefits everyone! Can you commit to a 'Tech-free Tuesday', or maybe a 'Fabulous Friday' where you focus on the positives from the week? Having an accountability buddy or group will support you in developing a healthy relationship with your digital media.

Figure 3.3 Useful strategies for managing the health of your digital diet

consider the following question: 'Do you need support to manage your tech use?' There are a variety of features that can help you achieve your own personal sense of digital well-being that will help you understand your technology use, disconnect when you can and thus create healthy habits that you would be able to share with not only your own family, but your patients and their surrounding families. The research by Gillaspy and Vasilica (2021) illustrates how taking these steps can have a positive impact.

> *Upon reflection . . . I realised . . . I set myself the challenge of having a minimum of one hour a day digital media free. Initially, this challenge failed . . . However, with perseverance I found this task becoming easier . . . Over time, I felt myself become less reliant on technology and I am feeling the health benefits . . . I've been able to connect on a deeper level with friends and family during technology free contact.*

As this activity is based on your own reflection, no answer is given at the end of this chapter.

Chapter summary

There is no question that social media, if used correctly as a professional, can be advantageous. Its far-reaching nature is a quick fix for healthcare professionals who are expected to keep up to date with the latest evidence-based research while working. Social media platforms can be used to push specific articles, papers or evidence-based research electronically. This is being seen more and more among academics who may follow researchers in their field. Social media can provide healthcare professionals a space to collaborate, share ideas, generate discussion and keep up to date with their own professional development. As you have seen in an earlier chapter within this book, there are many benefits to having a social media account, but consider the impact of social media platforms, working on assignments for long periods of time on your emotional well-being. As a healthcare professional, you have a duty of care to yourself, your patients and the profession you are registered to, to look after your own mental health. However, as you have read throughout this chapter, there are considerations that must be adhered to when considering your own professional position when using such platforms. If you are in any doubt, it would be wise to review your profession's viewpoint, policy or standards on the use of social media.

Activities: brief outline answers

Activity 3.1   Reflection (page 39)

You may want to begin by reflecting on digital technology and your own habits. Perhaps you could align these into positive and negative categories, and begin to reinforce and build upon those that you feel enhance your digital well-being. Consider how you could change your negative habits to protect your digital well-being.

Activity 3.2 Patient confidentiality and respect (page 40)

As a student nurse/nurse, you have a duty of care to protect the public. Both of the scenarios breach patient confidentiality and should be escalated. In both instances, it is vital to speak to somebody who is one of your practice supervisors, university tutor or ward manager. If the person breaching patient confidentiality is any of the above, the next step would be to escalate the issue to someone more senior – for instance, the head of school or matron. It could be suggested that making both the head of school and matron aware would be best practice.

Activity 3.3 Understanding your digital footprint (page 41)

Begin this activity by searching for yourself using a search engine and reflect on your image portrayed to the online community. Second, when thinking about ways in which to alter your digital footprint, you may begin to deactivate old accounts, unsubscribe from mailing lists and remember always to think before you post.

Activity 3.4 Reflection (page 44)

A useful starting point is to consider that the NMC stance is that nurses are accountable for maintaining professional boundaries with patients. If Emma were to accept the friend's request, could this result in a breach of this boundary with Susan? Consider that Emma's employer may have specific guidance on social media usage and, if Emma is unsure, she should also consult this. When considering alternatives, Emma's organisation may have a social media presence that Susan may wish to engage with rather than an individual staff member.

Activity 3.5 Reflection (page 45)

Locate your university Fitness to Practise policy and engage with this document. Reread the scenario within the chapter and consider the process that Rachel will now be required to engage with in terms of a reported FtP.

Activity 3.6 Reviewing clinical practice guidance (page 46)

Do the documents you regularly access within the clinical environment address the topic of cyberbullying? Begin to reflect on this important topic. Could you help champion addressing this issue within your clinical environment?

Useful websites

www.wecommunities.org

We Communities: a useful collection of Twitter chats run by healthcare professionals.

www.dsptoolkit.nhs.uk

NHS Digital Data Security and Protection Toolkit: supports organisations in identifying vulnerabilities and implementing plans to overcome any identified areas of high risk.

Chapter 4

Harnessing the potential of your digital collaborations

Lisa Garwood-Cross and Michael Haslam

HEE Digital Capabilities Framework

This chapter will address the following domains of digital capability:

Teaching, learning and self-development (level 2)

- Participate in online learning forums or communities (e.g., leave comments, respond to questions in forums)

Communication, collaboration and participation (level 2)

- Use a range of digital communication methods at personal and professional level and according to the purpose and audience needs
- Use a wide range of digital technologies to communicate and collaborate with people acting accordingly and appropriately
- Demonstrate and champion ethical, positive, sensitive and appropriate attitudes and behaviours in digital communication, collaboration and participation

Technical proficiency (level 2)

- Use a wide range of software and applications for personal and professional use both individually and with others

Chapter aims

After reading this chapter, you will be able to:

- understand the importance of digital collaborations in virtual spaces both for the benefit of others and your own personal development;

- be able to identify the benefits of Online Networked Communities (access to information, shared knowledge, feedback and better information workflows) and recognise the potential role of social media within these;
- be able to identify some potential challenges of online collaborations and have considered how you might navigate them.

Introduction

During your time as a nursing student and beyond, you will undoubtedly engage in digital collaborations, both academically and within clinical practice. This goes beyond the use of electronic patient records and emailing colleagues to include those tools discussed earlier in this book, such as cloud-based platforms for sharing documents and video-conferencing software to converse with colleagues and patients. This chapter focuses on working together in virtual spaces, both for the benefit of patients, and for your own personal and professional development. Using case studies and scenarios as illustrations, we discuss the benefits of digital collaborations to help you recognise the potential opportunities presented by working together in virtual spaces. The concept of digital professionalism within the context of your digital collaborations will also be explored towards the end of this chapter, some potential 'digital dilemmas' supporting you to navigate the potential challenges and issues that you might encounter while collaborating with others online.

Digital collaborations for the benefit of service users

Digital devices and virtual spaces provide many ways for people to come together and can be utilised in healthcare to increase collaboration between individuals and their care team or to create communities of peer support. In this section, we demonstrate how digital collaborations can be used in a multitude of ways to benefit a wide range of people, regardless of health condition or age. Activity 4.1 below demonstrates how a residential care home might use digital technologies to support collaborations for the benefit of their residents.

Activity 4.1   Reflection

A residential care home is looking to find ways to improve the well-being of their residents through the use of digital technology. They have invested in several new technologies.

1. An electronic care plan system to make linking up of care easier and to save staff time completing paperwork.

(Continued)

(Continued)

2. A large digital tablet table that acts as a sensory station to encourage fine motor skills through digital games.
3. Using Skype to video call families of residents who do not live in the local area to reduce social isolation.
4. A digital time capsule app for patients with dementia where photographs, memories and music from their life can be stored to aid with memory recognition.

Rate your confidence in using each of these technologies out of 5 (5-high confidence).

What skills would you like to develop to help you build confidence with these technologies?

As this activity is based on your own reflection, no outline answer is given at the end of this chapter.

There are a variety of ways above that show how technologies might be used to stimulate and engage service users in this setting, as well as increasing time-saving measures for staff. The variety of technologies available and their ability to be used, adapted and applied to different kinds of service users means that they can be useful across different health and social care contexts.

Digital collaborations can also benefit patients by supporting healthcare professionals to understand patient perspectives, which feed into the care that we provide. Virtual spaces allow us unprecedented access to publicly shared patient perspectives of certain health conditions and of using health services. Activity 4.2 below illustrates this.

Activity 4.2   Understanding patient perspectives

Many patients, especially those with chronic, rare or life-changing conditions use the internet and social media platforms to blog, post or create video blogs (vlogs) as an eHealth diary about their lived experiences with a condition. Patient eHealth diaries have been found to provide patients with a voice and create rich information for healthcare professionals (Wilson et al., 2016). One way to improve your quality of care is to take time to understand the lived experiences of patients through engaging with these resources online.

*   Choose a health condition and find a patient video blog or blog related to it.
*   You can search for blogs on Google, videos on YouTube, accounts on Instagram or any other social media platform.
*   Write down what it teaches you about patient lived experience and how you think this might be utilised to improve the care you deliver to others.

As this activity is based on your own reflection, no outline answer is given at the end of this chapter.

It is important, however, to note that when engaging with spaces where health service users are sharing their opinions, we must ensure that we remain impartial and professional. This might feel difficult if you are reading or watching someone criticise your local trust or your profession. We will discuss digital professionalism in more depth in the final section of this chapter.

Another way that virtual collaborations can benefit service users is through the development of patient communities. For some patients, particularly for those who have long-term conditions, illness can be a lonely experience. Therefore, patients may use the internet and social media to connect with other people with similar health conditions. These communities can become peer-support networks where patients share their experiences, support each other and engage socially with others who understand their condition (Dhar et al., 2018). Engaging with online patient communities has been found to have positive outcomes in long-term conditions (Merolli et al., 2013) and they have been used for a variety of health contexts, including mental health, cancer and chronic kidney disease.

Research summary: The Kidney Information Network

The Kidney Information Network (KIN) is a series of localised social media micro-communities providing peer support to patients with chronic kidney disease (CKD), enabling patients to network, create and share information with each other and with clinicians. KIN was created as a patient-centred intervention and works to initiate positive social change within the local renal community of patients. The community aspect of KIN centres around private patient-led Facebook groups that act as local micro-communities for CKD patients. However, the site also functions as a hub where patients can blog about their experiences and access information through other social media platforms such as YouTube and Twitter.

KIN users have self-organised collaborative question-and-answer sessions with healthcare professionals from their local trust to answer patient questions about renal diet, shielding during the COVID-19 pandemic and post-transplant recovery. These sessions were conducted via video-conferencing software Zoom, recorded and then shared onto the local KIN Facebook group for those unable to attend. Group members also created their own 'healthy choices' weight-loss accountability group with a local renal dietician that met remotely during the COVID-19 pandemic.

KIN has been found to benefit patients access to healthcare information, help patients feel more informed about their condition and positively contribute to the mental health of patients by providing a safe space to discuss frustrations and anxieties, and receive valuable support from peers (Vasilica et al., 2020, 2021).

The Kidney Information Network in the Research Summary example above shows how social media can be harnessed to connect patients with each other. Alongside providing peer support, The Kidney Information Network also brought together healthcare providers and patients in a new and innovative way, providing easily accessible information and access to support outside conventional times and places, particularly during the COVID-19 pandemic.

Harnessing your online collaborations to support your own development

Collaboration within virtual spaces can support your learning, helping you develop academic skills and even, as a qualified nurse, increase your opportunities for Continued Professional Development (CPD). In this section, we discuss the benefits of online networked communities, including those via social media, to develop knowledge and critical thinking skills. We will also consider how being a member of online communities may contribute to the development of your professional identity.

Case study: the online journal club

At the height of the COVID-19 pandemic, Liz and her friend Amelia felt isolated from their classmates as many classes were taking place online. To combat this, Liz and Amelia started a weekly informal coffee club to meet with classmates outside the virtual classroom via Microsoft Teams and felt this helped them feel connected, especially during their placement.

Alongside this, in preparation for their upcoming assignment, Liz and Amelia organised a fortnightly journal club, taking turns to present and critique papers. The students felt this online collaboration supported their classroom learning and continued the online journal club even after face-to-face learning resumed. Liz and Amelia feel the benefits of these online collaborations go beyond mutual support, by developing reflection and critical analysis skills that helped them to obtain higher marks in their assignments.

The case study above illustrates how online networked communities can provide peer support and is an example of how virtual collaborations can provide opportunities to further develop the academic and practical skills and knowledge necessary for nursing. Technology that supported the continuation of nurse education during the pandemic can, if harnessed correctly, continue to be a key instrument for collaboration and communication throughout your education and beyond. Although the platforms that nursing students use may vary due to institution and learner preference, there are benefits to engaging and collaborating with each other virtually. The NMC (2019) encourages the use of online networked communities to a) access resources relevant for

CPD, b) support the building of professional relationships and c) to engage with other healthcare professionals globally.

The benefits of networked communities via social media

If you use social media, you likely already engage, or have engaged, with online networked communities with peers, friends, family and work colleagues using platforms such as WhatsApp, Facebook, Snapchat, Instagram, TikTok and Twitter. They can range from formal communities set up by your university, using institution-approved platforms, to the WhatsApp group used to communicate informally around course issues with your peers.

Online networked communities are usually formed by and around the use of open and closed online groups to which members are added. Other platforms such as the microblogging site, Twitter, use identifiable 'hashtags' such as #WeStNs and #WeNurses to group text and posts together, allowing people to engage in conversation with others around their common interests and practice, facilitating the sharing of knowledge. Regardless of platform (our intention here is not to discuss the nuances, benefits and challenges of engagement, as your engagement will depend upon your task and preferred platform), the immediate benefits of online networked communities include the currency and accessibility of information across both time and geographical boundaries.

Online networked communities, especially those via social media, can become valuable learning tools if used in a professional capacity (Haslam, 2020), the potential benefits increasing as the user steps to new levels of participation (Figure 4.1).

1. At the most basic level, online networked communities allow users to curate information, staying up to date with news and the evidence base relevant to their specialism. Users at this level may prefer to observe others 'lurking' in the background, or may superficially interact with online networks by following or 'liking' others posts.

2. Beyond this, users may begin increasing their interactions with others online, commenting on or sharing others' posts. Here, users start to connect with others and become involved in the exchange of ideas around healthcare issues.

3. At the highest level, users may actively engage with online networked communities through the creation of content and posts for the purpose of initiating discussions. At this level, professional networking opportunities are increased and debate is enabled, with users sharing best practice and becoming involved in a shared discourse around current healthcare issues.

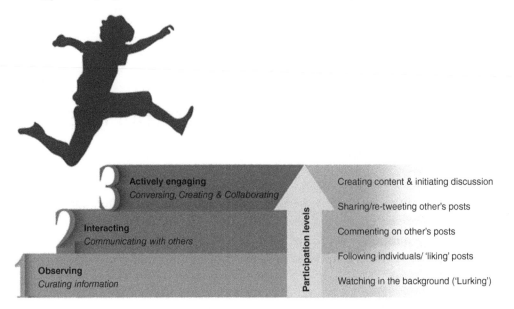

Figure 4.1   The steps of online engagement

You may find the diagram above useful as a way of reflecting upon your own levels of engagement in the different online networked communities within which you already participate. The potential benefits of active engagement and participation in online networked communities, especially those via social media, are listed in Table 4.1 with examples, and are aligned with Beckingham's '6Cs' model (Beckingham, 2019).

Online networked communities via social media may empower users to become:		
Curators	• Knowledge is easily accessed, free of charge. • The user is kept up to date with the latest information, policy and shifting evidence-base.	*Example:* *Saving a post with useful updates on policy or evidence to return to later.*
Communicators	• Promotes exchange of ideas and the sharing of best practice. • Encourages a clear and concise communication style as information must be carefully selected.	*Example:* *Responding to a post on the NMC NHS NURSES-UK Facebook group.*
Conversationalists	• Debate is enabled as users are exposed to and engage in a shared discourse around contemporary issues in healthcare. • Supporting the shift of users from passive recipients of information to active participants who can contribute to and drive the changing discourse around nursing issues.	*Example:* *Participating in a discussion within a private Facebook group for nursing students from your university.*

Online networked communities via social media may empower users to become:		
Collaborators	• Engagement with professionals and experts across boundaries of geography, time and with some platforms, hierarchy. • Facilitating supportive peer and professional networks. • Also strengthens connections to the higher education institution, practice and the wider community. • Promotes professional networking that may increase future employment opportunities.	*Example:* *Being able to connect with a head of nursing through a #WeNurses tweetchat.*
Creators	• Encourages the creation of content, allowing ideas to be quickly disseminated and knowledge shared.	*Example:* *Creating a short TikTok video with tips for other nursing students on getting the most out of their placements.*
Critics	• Critical analytical skills are improved through information selection and interrogation. • Critical thinking is an essential skill for nurses and Activity 4.3 at the end of this chapter will support you with the development of your critical thinking skills when interrogating online sources.	*Example:* *Watching a YouTube video about a procedure and assessing if it contains reliable information and best practice.*

Table 4.1 Benefits of participating in online networked communities with examples

For nursing students, active participation in online networked communities may provide additional benefits to those listed in the table above; virtual communities of practice also support the development of professional identities and socialisation into the nursing role.

Professional identity and virtual communities of practice

As nurses, we already engage in multiple physical communities, participating in the shared social practices of our academic and healthcare teams for the benefit of our patients and our own development. Lave and Wenger's (1991) model of situated learning is a useful theoretical framework here, proposing that the novice's legitimate interactions with those with more expertise within our communities supports the development of their knowledge and skills.

For nurses, this model is important, as it also provides a context for understanding the development of professional identities. As a nursing student, your active participation in the social and cultural practices of a group or *community of practice* (such as university or your clinical placements) mean that eventually, you too will become an experienced member of the team or community and in turn, one day support novice community members (such as students or junior staff). For these spaces to be identified as communities of practice, they must include a *community* of active members who *participate in learning* or *practice* within a *shared domain of interest*, as in Figure 4.2.

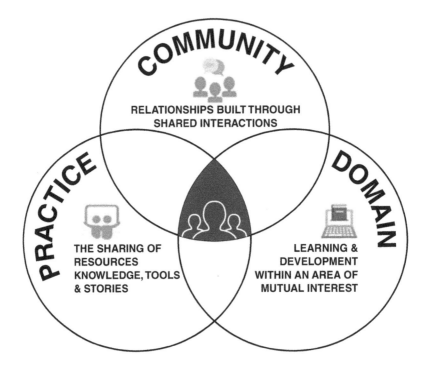

Figure 4.2 Communities of practice

Outside of the traditional boundaries of classroom walls and clinical placements, online networked spaces may also serve as communities of practice (Haslam, 2020), provided that community members are participating in learning within a shared domain of interest, such as that related to their specialism. The earlier research summary discussing the 'Kidney Information Network' is an example of how networked online communities can evolve into virtual communities of practice. While group members may begin with peripheral participation as novices, interactions with local healthcare practitioners and experienced group members contribute to the novice's knowledge acquisition and increase self-confidence in the management of their own condition, allowing them, in turn, to become experts by experience.

Personal and professional growth are linked to the active participation in the social practices of these communities. This is because virtual communities of practice also offer the chances for instant feedback, providing opportunities for self-reflection. This is a dynamic process, where the self is constantly negotiated and renegotiated, impacting upon the individual's thoughts, attitudes and behaviours. Therefore, participation in online spaces can also support the development of your professional identity and socialisation into the nursing role.

Digital professionalism: examining your digital collaborations

This chapter has, so far, focused upon the benefits of collaborations online within virtual spaces. As you enter the nursing profession, however, it is important that you exercise caution when collaborating online as the utilisation of public social media platforms in particular may have professional implications if they are not used appropriately. The final section of this chapter asks you to consider how you present yourself online and to reduce your role in the spread of misinformation by interrogating the credibility of sources of information.

Your 'digital footprint'

In Chapter 3, you were invited to explore your digital footprint, but it is important to examine this again here within the context of your online collaborations. Once anything you share online is in the public domain, it becomes a part of your digital footprint and as it is easily shared or downloaded by others, may be difficult to erase. In a world where even temporary posts such as Snapchat stories can be captured by screenshot, anything you share online should therefore be treated as potentially public and permanent.

As you become aware of how your actions online may be perceived by others, it can feel challenging at first to navigate the boundaries around how you participate in virtual spaces. However, an understanding of how you present yourself online is key to the development of your online professional identity (Beckingham, 2019) and reduces the risk of professional reputations being tarnished by unprofessional behaviour online. Luckily, the NMC provides guidance around this (NMC, 2019) and a wealth of videos on the responsible use of social media and online professionalism are available via their website (NMC.org.uk).

What are you communicating?

The features on social media platforms can make sharing content a two-second task, but it is useful to take a moment before posting to consider what you are communicating to others. You might ask yourself, 'Is there any way someone might misunderstand my intention?' You should also consider how different shorthand phrases, slang or text speak might mean different things to different people and, if in doubt, it is better to avoid using these. For example, the acronym 'LOL' can commonly be interpreted as either 'laughing out loud' or 'lots of love', potentially leading to offensive miscommunication between people when their interpretations of this acronym are different.

It is also important to think of what you may be communicating to others before you 'like' or share a 'status' or post that is not created by you and consider the potential implications of doing so. Consider the case study below.

Case study: Toni and Jenny

Toni and Jenny are first-year nursing students and previously worked as healthcare support workers together before starting university and being placed in the same clinical area. Toni added Jenny as a friend on Facebook so they could communicate with and support each other outside of work.

In the past two weeks, however, Toni has had an issue with her academic assessor and has taken to her social media accounts to voice her unhappiness with her placement and the clinical area in general. In her most recent post, she made a passing comment in the post to mistreatment of patients, tagging Jenny into the post. Although Jenny had not witnessed this and did not believe it to be true, she felt obliged to 'like' the post to show support for Toni.

This case demonstrates how 'liking' a comment or being tagged into content may increase the risk of being linked with discussions or online content that are potentially contentious. Engaging with content in this way risks you being affiliated with, or seemingly endorsing, content that may not necessarily represent your own views. Within nursing, regardless of the stage of your career, you are required to uphold the reputation of your profession at all times, while also understanding how your actions might influence others (NMC, 2018a). The NMC therefore advises considering who and what you associate with on social media as being mentioned in posts that are inappropriate may put your professional reputation at risk (NMC, 2019).

The blurring of boundaries

It is important that people maintain their digital and ethical integrity in virtual spaces. However, there are times when the boundaries between the private and professional in virtual spaces may become blurred, leading individuals to forget that their conduct should be maintained to the same standards as face-to-face interactions, as seen in the scenario below.

Scenario: connecting with work colleagues online

You are part of a work WhatsApp group for a role that involves the care of vulnerable young people. In the group chat, several colleagues express frustrations about a difficult patient in your care. Some of the messages sent by your colleagues refer to the patient as an 'f***ing idiot' and state they 'wish he'd f*** off'.

Activity 4.3 Reflection

From the scenario above:

• How would you navigate this situation?
• What do you think could have been done differently by the people involved to use this resource as a positive professional support tool?

As this activity is based on your own reflection, no outline answer is given at the end of this chapter.

While we are all aware of patient rights to privacy online in that we should not share confidential information inappropriately or post photographs of people in receipt of our care online without their prior and informed consent, the right to the respect of the people in your care should also be extended to online spaces, even in a situation where you believe you have complete anonymity. This includes inappropriate comments about patients, bullying, discrimination, intimidation, encouragement of violence or inciting hatred.

Misinformation

While virtual spaces and networked communities can help you to develop your skills as a nurse and expose you to best practice, they also require a critical eye. Social media can be a useful source of information and expose you to current debates within healthcare, but online content is not always regulated and so may also be a source of misinformation. This is an issue, as any information or advice you share via social networks must be evidence based and correct to the best of your knowledge according to the NMC *Code* (NMC, 2018a). Consider the scenario below.

Scenario: Margaret

While sitting by the bedside of Margaret, one of your patients, she tells you that she has been offered the COVID-19 vaccination, but discloses that she doesn't want to accept it as she has heard on Facebook that it is a government conspiracy to 'control the masses'.

Margaret is 54, a smoker and has been admitted to hospital with a respiratory illness. She hasn't got COVID-19 but has been struggling to breathe prior to admission. She has heard from friends on Facebook that COVID-19's symptoms are no worse than those of a common cold.

(Continued)

(Continued)

- Regardless of your own views, how might you have dealt with this situation?
- Consider the social media content that you have 'liked' or shared in the past? What messages might you have inadvertently communicated to others?

Having a critical eye, and so the ability to interrogate the credibility of sources, would not only ensure that you are confident in identifying misinformation, but would also prepare you for encountering patients, such as Margaret, who may have formed opinions based on misinformation. Remember, critical thinking in nursing is an essential skill and taking a little extra time to interrogate the credibility of sources can also stop you from being part of the chain of misinformation and help you to prepare counter arguments to support your discussions with patients (Kata, 2012). This supports the NMC proficiency around thinking critically and drawing upon current evidence to make evidence-based decisions (NMC, 2018b). Our final activity of this chapter, Activity 4.4 below, may help you to do this.

Activity 4.4   Source credibility

YouTube is a growing source of health information, particularly with young people. The 2020 Digital Health Generation report with English young people aged 11–18 found that YouTube was the most popular source of health information, with almost half of survey respondents reporting use (Rich et al., 2020). YouTube can also be used in your professional practice to explore best practice, develop your learning in bite-size chunks, understand patient perspectives and to share resources with patients. However, as with any platform where users can create content, not all health information on YouTube is accurate, and misinformation can easily be disseminated.

Using the same health condition you selected for Activity 4.2 earlier in this chapter, go to the YouTube website or app and search for the health condition. As you scroll through the results and click on videos, use the checklist below to assess the video:

- Who created and posted the video? Does it appear to be a reputable source?
- What type of content is this – an educational video, a lecture, a patient vlog, a television clip, etc.?
- When was the video posted? Is it still up to date and relevant, and has the creator posted an updated video if it is several years old?
- Is the content evidence based and an example of best practice?
- Do you feel this is accurate information or misinformation?
- How has the public response of the video been received? How many views, likes or dislikes has it received and what do the comments say?

Reflect on your investigations and consider if misinformation is better or worse received than evidence-based information? How does this help you support your patients in making informed choices about their health?

As this activity is based on your own reflection, no answer is given at the end of this chapter.

Chapter summary

As we bring this chapter to a close, please be assured that the aim of this final discussion around digital professionalism and the challenges when collaborating online is not to alarm you and to put you off collaborating with others in virtual spaces. Instead, it is hoped that the case studies and scenarios here have given you an opportunity to reflect upon your own digital collaborations and to sharpen your critical thinking, thus preparing you to become a skilled digital collaborator in any virtual environment. We hope that this chapter has highlighted the value of digital collaborations and their potential to both improve the care delivered to service users and support your own development and socialisation into the nursing role. Once successfully navigated, online networked communities can promote a dynamic learning experience and become powerful tools for professional development.

Useful website

www.kinet.site

The Kidney Information Network (KIN) provides peer support to patients with chronic kidney disease, enabling them to network, create and share information with each other and with clinicians.

Chapter 5

Unleashing your digital creativity to enhance person-centred care

(with special acknowledgement to the Comensus group at the University of Central Lancashire)

Janet Garner and Steph Holmes

HEE Digital Capabilities Framework

This chapter will address the following domains of digital capability:

Creation, innovation and research (level 2)

- Use digital technologies to curate or create new ideas, methods, solutions and decisions

Communication, collaboration and participation (level 2)

- Use a wide range of digital technologies to communicate and collaborate with people acting accordingly and appropriately
- Demonstrate and champion ethical, positive, sensitive and appropriate attitudes and behaviours in digital communication, collaboration and participation

Teaching, learning and self-development (level 2)

- Seek appropriate and innovative digital technologies to enhance learning for self and others

Technical proficiency (level 2)

- Use a wide range of software and applications for personal and professional use both individually and with others

Chapter aims

After reading this chapter, you will be able to:

- explore the creation and co-creation of digital content for service users, carers, patients and their families;
- consider the impact that digital technology has had on communications with service users, carers, patients and their families, and the impact it has had on nurses and the nursing profession;
- examine the limitations and barriers, both technological and social, of digital engagement for patients and families and ways in which these limitations can be overcome.

Motivate healthcare professionals to be leaders in digital creativity.

Introduction

Having digital technologies is brilliant. When Dad was more able, having Tapo cameras in his living room, bedroom and kitchen assured me he was safe and I was able to call him on Facebook if I saw him doing something dangerous or if he had forgotten to do something.

Online support group has been so positive in understanding my partner's condition, supporting others, and identifying with other carers.

(*State of Caring*, Carers UK, 2021)

Person- and family-centred care and enhanced communication skills have become a key focus of professional health and social care education in recent years (NMC, 2018a). In addition, there has been a fundamental shift in the rhetoric and delivery of care from 'doing to you' to 'working with you'. This shift towards shared decision-making and co-creation of improvements and changes in the way that nurses engage with people can be seen in the ways that service users, carers and patients are increasingly involved in the education and training of student nurses, as well as the co-design of services and the development of new digital content for different audiences. In this chapter, we will share some of our experiences of creating content, as well as reflect on some of the barriers and enablers in seeking to create effective content for service users, carers, patients and their families.

A note on terminology

Within this chapter, we refer to people in receipt of health and social care services as service users, carers, patients and families. During your studies or professional career, you may also encounter other terms such as 'people with lived experience'. We also refer to the 'Comensus group' (our service user and carer group at the University of Central Lancashire), Comensus 'members' and 'volunteers' (as service users and carers often do not receive payment for their involvement). Carers in the UK are defined as 'anyone who cares, unpaid, for a friend or family member who due to illness, disability, a mental health problem or an addiction cannot cope without their support' (Carers Trust, 2015). Depending on your own field, you may use different terminology to describe members of the public who seek to be involved in their own care, in supporting others or in helping co-design service improvements. Care must be taken to check with the person or people involved of course, by *asking the individual* how they would like to be referred to.

Usability and accessibility of digital materials

The idea of digital engagement has seen a steady growth over the past twenty years, but in March 2020 it was given a sudden and unexpected urgency in the UK with the emergence of SARS-CoV-2 or Covid-19. Suddenly, the need to explore non-contact ways of communicating became very urgent, and person-centred care was perhaps forgotten in the rush to create digital content and digital engagement for patients and professionals, with little initial thought that this might disenfranchise a large section of the population.

A more measured approach eventually prevailed with a return to person-centred care and consideration about how users would engage with digital content.

Initially, most digital content was static, transferring existing documents and procedures to the digital realm and creating new static documents to mimic existing systems and processes. Those users who could, engaged with this static content by simply accessing it on the internet, but the authors then had to consider how users might engage with richer and more dynamic content.

The creation of digital content, rather than simply accessing documents, required thought into the tools and methods available, and this created a whole new set of problems. To be universally useful, a digital resource needs to be update-able by many different people with many different skill sets, and training on these tools also needs to be delivered universally and accessibly. Additional issues arise when a resource has to be updated by many different people, leading to conflicts.

Box 5.1   Electronic patient records

Excellent examples of online resources and documentation that needs to be kept updated by multiple people are the EMIS system in use by Clinical Commissioning Groups (CCGs) and the RiO system that Lancashire and South Cumbria Foundation Trust use for Electronic Patient Records. The EMIS system in particular needs to be accessed by people of all skill levels, from receptionists making notes of upcoming appointments to health professionals (including nurses) entering complex medical information about the patient. Furthermore, there is a requirement under NHS information governance confidentiality guidelines to ensure that the information is only seen by those authorised to do so. This is a prime example of a many-to-many system whereby entirely different sets of people are allowed to make alterations to those allowed to see the information, including personal access by individual patients to their own NHS records.

Access to digital resources has become more complex with the multiplicity of devices available now and their radically different capabilities, all of which have to be taken into account when designing the resource. Will images that are clear when viewed on a desktop computer be usable on a mobile phone? Is your content usable by those with adaptive technologies such as screen readers? What price is your fancy graphic when it needs a fast internet connection to download and a lot of users are still on Dial-up or mobile communication?

The UK Government has a set of standards about the size of internet pages and speed of access which could well be adopted across the whole area of digital accessibility. As an aside, services with optimised front-end performance are also better for the environment because they use less power. And since users do not have to upgrade their devices as often to keep up with performance demands, fewer devices get thrown away.

Case study: creating the Chrysalis Transexual Support Group's website

The Chrysalis Transexual Support Group's website is an example of speed leading the design. Chrysalis is an unfunded community organisation that gives support and advocacy to young and old trans people throughout the North of England. Each page of the website is designed to load quickly and give links to other more complex information in both summary and complete form. There is an indication that the complete page may take some time to download, giving the user the choice to, for instance, download the summary page now and the complete page when attached to a Wi-Fi router. This also overcomes the technical problems associated with updating large and complex pages, but one has to ensure that the summary and complete pages remain synchronised. To date, the website has been accessed by over 3,500 people. Is this testimony to its currency and usability? Please see the World Wide Web consortium usability standards and Jakob Nielsen's 10 principles to find out more about how to ensure that online content is usable:

- www.w3.org/standards
- www.nngroup.com/articles/ten-usability-heuristics

Co-creating digital content with the public

Service user and carer involvement in education and services

The main driver for the full integration of service user and carer involvement in professional education is to target and prevent future failings in care such as those uncovered in the Francis Report (Francis, 2013) by placing an emphasis on a compassionate, person-centred approach to care (Scammell, 2017).

Service user and carer involvement in education and healthcare services, however, is not a new development in the UK or indeed across the world. Systematic reviews of involvement in higher education have highlighted the growth in this area since the beginning of this century (Robinson and Webber, 2013; Scammell et al., 2016; Towle et al., 2010) and focused on the benefits to service users, carers and students alike. Their involvement is not limited to teaching and learning. Increasingly, public stakeholders with lived experience of services are invited to contribute to curriculum design, course approval meetings, admissions events and assessment (Scammell et al., 2016). Healthcare education policy in the UK has moved on from 'recommending' involvement to 'requiring' the involvement of real-life experiences in the curriculum and the 'co-production' of curricula (NMC, 2018b) in their standards for education. Hopefully, you will have had the benefit of real-life experience delivered by a member of the public in your own education or training, and experienced first-hand the impact it can have on your personal and professional development. You may not have been aware of the breadth of involvement *behind the scenes* in recruitment discussions, course approval meetings and curriculum design.

Principles of co-production and co-creation in Higher Education and services

We have already mentioned one of the current policy drivers that has helped drive co-production in healthcare education. Examples of others include the Health and Care Professions Council (HCPC) who regulate a number of allied health professions and courses such as Paramedic Science, Occupational Therapy and Physiotherapy, Social Work England, the General Medical Council and the General Pharmaceutical Council, to name but a few. All these regulators now stipulate that people must be involved in the programme. Some go further than others and mention specific areas, but we must acknowledge that this change in ideology has not occurred overnight. The emergence of social movements such as the feminist movement and anti-war agenda of the 1960s, the consumer rights movement in the 1970s and 1980s, and Disability Rights in the 1980s and 1990s, all contributed to what many sociologists see as a shift in the balance of power between public service provider or professional, and the service user or patient. The rise of the service-user movement in nursing began in the mental health field where there were many accusations of paternalism, a general withholding of rights and feelings of having no power to influence their own lives. The Patient's Charter (Department of Health, 1991) defined patients as consumers with rights for the first time and has led to subsequent incremental changes over the years that followed.

Nursing and Midwifery Council: co-production and co-creation

The Nursing and Midwifery Council and NHS are now encouraging co-production and co-creation in the design of all services and education for health professionals.

> *Co-production acknowledges that people with 'lived experience' of a particular condition are often best placed to advise on what support and services will make a positive difference to their lives. Done well, co-production helps to ground discussions in reality, and to maintain a person-centred perspective.*

(Coalition for Personalised Care)

Figure 5.1 illustrates the four principles of co-production outlined by the Social Care Institute for Excellence. It is imperative, therefore, when thinking about designing any new service, digital or in-person, that the principles of co-production and co-creation are included in your planning.

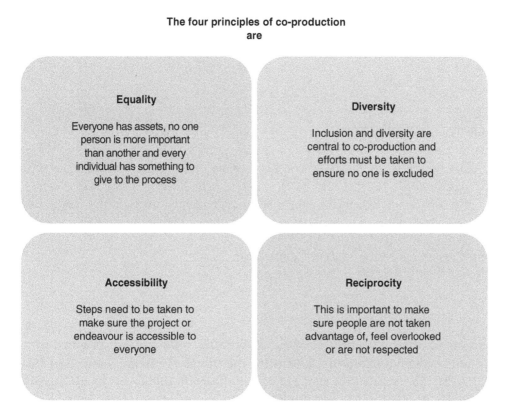

The four principles of co-production are

Equality

Everyone has assets, no one person is more important than another and every individual has something to give to the process

Diversity

Inclusion and diversity are central to co-production and efforts must be taken to ensure no one is excluded

Accessibility

Steps need to be taken to make sure the project or endeavour is accessible to everyone

Reciprocity

This is important to make sure people are not taken advantage of, feel overlooked or are not respected

Figure 5.1 Four principles of co-production (adapted from the Social Care Institute for Excellence [www.scie.org.uk/publications/guides/guide51/what-is-coproduction/principles-of-coproduction.asp], accessed 1 November 2021)

Case study: Comensus

The Comensus (Community Engagement and Service User support) group was set up as a resource for nurse education in 2004 at the University of Central Lancashire, UK (Mckeown et al., 2010). The group is made up of over 100 volunteers with mental health or physical health conditions or who are carers for friends and family members. Most members live in the local area and are currently using local health and social care services. Their involvement has traditionally taken place face-to-face, with students and lecturers in classrooms and meeting rooms. All participants value this approach as it promotes personal engagement and often builds a direct emotional connection between the service user or carer and the student nurse. Service users and carers have the opportunity to 'see' their audience in real time and students are able to interact with service users and carers in a 'safe' environment. It is an example of co-production in health education.

The growth in demand for NHS nurses, however, has led to an increase in student numbers and satellite campuses at our university, and this has had an impact on the finite numbers (and time) of Comensus members and their ability to meet the demand for their input. It is suggested by managers that Comensus members film their stories and experiences instead, thus freeing up their time and allowing members to focus on other projects.

Activity 5.1   Reflection

1. How do you think the service users and carers from Comensus might react to this suggestion?
2. What do you think the impact would be on students and learners of this change in the method of delivery of personal experiences?

An outline answer is provided at the end of this chapter.

Comensus volunteers co-produced a collaborative reflection on practice with students and academics exploring lessons for the future of nursing education (Garner et al., 2022). The words shown in Figure 5.2 illustrate the keywords we used in our collaborative conversations when describing the future of authentic digitally enabled nursing education.

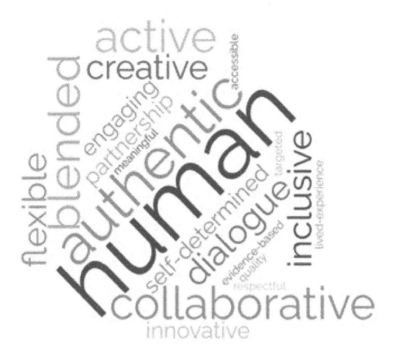

Figure 5.2   Co-creating the future of digitally enabled nursing education

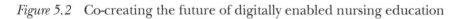

Research summary: co-production principles

Read more about general co-production principles and the benefits of involving people in the development of new services or projects via these sites:

- Social Care Institute for Excellence: www.scie.org.uk/publications/guides/guide51/
- Nursing and Midwifery Council blog: What co-production means to me: www.nmc.org.uk/news/news-and-updates/blog-nothing-about-me-without-me-the-value-of-co-production/
- Nursing and Midwifery Council Standards Framework for nursing education: www.nmc.org.uk/globalassets/sitedocuments/standards-of-proficiency/standards-framework-for-nursing-and-midwifery-education/education-framework.pdf
- The report here adds more depth into co-production (especially in mental health): https://strenco.eu/output-3-ways-of-working http://usir.salford.ac.uk/id/eprint/62541/1/Output%203%20report%20inc%20data%20analysis.pdf

Communicating in the digital age: a person-centred approach

There are now many means of communicating digitally, such as Skype, Zoom, Microsoft Teams, GoTo Meeting, StarLeaf, Cisco Webex, etc. There are social media sites, such as LinkedIn, Twitter, Facebook, TikTok and Instagram, and these all bring an opportunity to communicate with patients and the public in new ways. As nurses and health professionals, you are in a powerful position and can utilise new technologies to send public health messages to your patients and carers, as well as seek their help in co-designing improvements.

For example, in July 2021 a new app was launched by the CHAMPS Public Health Collaborative in Merseyside, UK, called 'Lower my Drinking', which enables service users to manage their own alcohol use and use online tools to reduce harmful levels of alcohol. See the list of Useful websites at the end of the chapter for more information about this campaign and app.

Another new digital resource was launched in 2022, Alcohol Licensing Community (alcohollicensing.org.uk), following research with residents to help the local community to raise any concerns relating to alcohol licensing in their area. A website can be used to store multimedia resources and also host a blog for service user and carer views and feedback. When you are considering decision making, consider different ways you can involve your service users, carers and their families; you can even create an infographic to help you communicate in a creative way (see Figure 5.3 as an example).

Scenario

You are employed within a GP practice and have been asked to help the nurse practitioner design a new digital service promoting 'Walking for Well-being'. The proven benefits of walking on mental and physical health are now widely documented, but this message does not seem to be reaching your local patient population.

Activity 5.2 Digital co-creativity

Reading the scenarios above:

As a new member of the multidisciplinary team, you are keen to impress. What steps could you take to consider the design of a new online resource for patients and their families? What would you want to include? Are there any particular social media sites you are familiar with? Are there any concerns from staff and patients that need to be addressed?

An outline answer is provided at the end of this chapter.

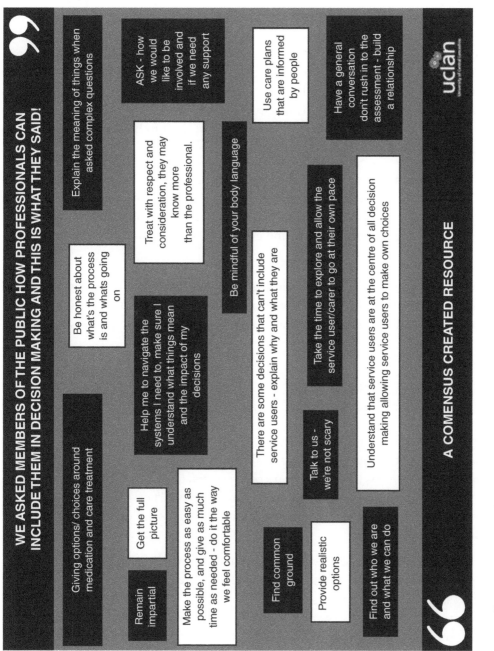

Figure 5.3 A Comensus-created resource for professional healthcare students (with special acknowledgement to Steven Seymour and Comensus for permission to use this image)

Cameras off or on?

The question of whether people have their cameras off or on during video calls has been a key debate from the increased use of such technologies since the global coronavirus pandemic. On one hand, since video technology in its simplest form just replaces face-to-face meetings, the use of a camera is an extension of that meeting and may be required to ensure that the person you are talking to is indeed the person that they say they are. The other side of the debate says that privacy and confidentiality issues arise when using video communication in certain settings – for instance, the home. Certainly, cameras are mandatory in many scenarios where professional intercommunication takes place, such as discussions with medical professionals, and are required in teaching sessions where the student is required to be professional, such as nursing or pharmacology.

There are clear advantages to using full video communication when it comes to telehealth. Your GP can see the problem area rather than rely on a spoken description over the telephone. There is no risk of passing on a contagion and there is also the opportunity to observe visual cues, which often become even more important within a mental health scenario.

This, however, requires that both service users and medical professionals be trained and at ease with visual communication, and be aware of any confidentiality issues. Seeing yourself on camera can be a daunting prospect, for professionals and patients alike.

Box 5.2   Unleashing digital creativity in education

In 2020, the global coronavirus pandemic and long lockdowns led to many changes in the way we live. In addition, our normal ways of working and studying were thrown into chaos by being unable to access the university spaces or equipment. Many health and social care staff and students were advised to work from home, while we know that many other staff and students were involved on the frontline fighting the effects of Covid-19 in exhausting and traumatic environments.

During these lockdowns, however, we adopted a different approach with the help of a fantastic digital learning service at our university. In 2019, Comensus had already created a digital resource library, which consists of service users' and carers' video case studies and written accounts which were created to support and enhance academic teaching. These are invaluable in providing resources across multi sites and modules. However, these 2D resources provide a challenge in that students can't interact with video case studies, so we developed a three-step plan in order to maintain involvement in our courses remotely. The list below demonstrates some of the digital resources we utilised during lockdown and will continue to embed in nursing curricula.

Microsoft Teams, also referred to as Teams, is a unified communication and collaboration platform that allows you to share files, video call, add in other applications and more. At Comensus, we used it for our volunteers to engage in live teaching events, consultations and simulated environments with students. We were also able to create a community where Comensus members can share what they are up to, connect with each other and attend a weekly drop-in where we all get on a video call and have a brew and a chat.

Padlet helps you to create content boards, add comments, pictures, links, videos etc. The best part is multiple people can view and interact with the document without needing a login. We have used the platform to generate content about the work we are doing and create an online business card for our community groups to connect and work together.

Flip allows the user to generate video discussions on a topic by creating grids for varying content areas and questions. We used Flip to pose questions to Comensus members – for example, about their lives during lockdown, asking them to provide a 'video diary' response. These teaching resources were very well received by students and enabled a vital way for students to continue to hear from the public while they are not on placement.

Finally, our volunteers still engage with us on the phone and by email. This means that they can be conferenced into meetings on the phone or computer, write new teaching resources and film themselves from home. All this work would not be possible without the hard work, dedication and commitment that our public members show the university, its staff and students.

Activity 5.3 Barriers and enablers to digital creativity

Health Education England (2018) have defined digital capability as 'those capabilities that fit someone for living, working, participating and thriving in a digital society'. For those involved with educating future professionals and designing health and social care curricula (including service users and carers), it is clear that content relating to digital education and the development of digital skills is vital to the future success of professional partnerships with patients and families. In an integrative review of nurses' digital capabilities (Brown et al., 2020), a key factor for nurses was self-reporting their skills as below average (Hwang and Park, 2011) or only slightly above competent (Kleib and Nagle, 2018). A negative correlation was noted between increasing age and skills competence also, with more mature nurses acknowledging a lack of digital training in their school and nursing education (Brown et al., 2020). However, the benefits of using digital technologies and being able to access electronic patient records are very clear in the embodiment of person-centred care, especially when service users, patients and carers are also empowered and trained in digital skills.

(Continued)

(Continued)

There are many barriers to digital engagement, and not least is that of training. People may have the requisite technology at home, but are unable to access digital resources because of a lack of support and guidance. Given a willingness to learn, this is relatively easy to overcome. The difficulty comes when the person has the technology but is unwilling to invest the required time or energy to learn the technology. It may be time constraints or physical constraints to accessing the training. One major problem is those people who do not have the requisite technology and may not be in a position to purchase that technology. This can be alleviated by the provision of devices to those people along with the necessary training.

An outline answer is provided at the end of this chapter.

Box 5.3 Encouraging engagement in university teaching by providing access to technology

Problem: In March 2020, few higher education staff and service user/carer members were using the full extent of digital capabilities and systems that their universities had to offer – for meetings, interviewing and teaching. At the University of Central Lancashire, Comensus members had previously been offered university IT accounts, which gave them access to university systems such as Outlook email and the Microsoft Office suite of software. Some of our Comensus volunteers were reasonably confident with IT and it was relatively straightforward to talk these people through the process over the telephone. Other members lacked the devices necessary to engage digitally and did not have Wi-Fi in their home.

Solution: We approached our colleagues at the University for financial and IT support for tablets and WiFi access and Comensus staff trained members in the use of both. All members were offered a personal one-to-one phone call to set them up and ensure they could download relevant applications. This approach worked well for Comensus and has been done at very little cost as spending could be offset against the reduction in travel costs.

Members were then given training in the use of digital technology. Doing this remotely presented problems, as it is no use telling people who don't know how to use Teams to access instructions for its use on Teams. The solution in many cases was first to contact the user by telephone to talk them through installation and initial set-up and then, once contact by Teams had been established, to go on to more complex instructions. In most cases, this worked well and continues to this day, with some users remaining online while others have re-engaged physically, adopting a 'blended approach'.

This still left a sizable group of volunteers who were not willing to engage digitally through personal choice. Instead, they agreed to be contacted only when the team returned to campus-based delivery.

Try to avoid making assumptions about age, social group, culture, etc. with regard to digital capability and access. For example, there is a common assumption that older people will have greater difficulty using technology, with the term 'digital natives' often used in media to describe younger generations who are more 'tech savvy'. However, this myth has now been widely debunked (Kirschner and Bruyckere, 2017) with the reverse of this often being true, as older people can have a wider experience of more aspects of technology, where younger people may be more expert but only in limited areas – social media, for instance. For example, 'I [Steph] am 69 with a degree in Computer Science and consider myself to be highly digitally capable'.

Case study: Mabel

An excellent example of assumptions being challenged happened to the mother of a friend of mine who became a resident in a social care home during the early stages of the pandemic. 'Mabel' is 103 years old and, apart from frailty issues, is entirely capable. As the care home was completely locked down, an alternative means had to be found to maintain contact between Mabel and her relatives. Although initially she had never used technology, she was introduced to the use of a Tablet and the Zoom platform, which she fully embraced, leading to a distinct upturn in her general mood and mental health. Indeed, in some cases Mabel preferred the electronic contact because 'she could simply turn off Zoom when she had had enough'.

There are initiatives afoot to improve the outcomes for the older generation which have been embraced wholeheartedly by the public. Many services moved to digital provision during the Covid-19 pandemic and, of course, this had an immense impact on the care and support given to service users and carers. The *State of Caring* report (Carers UK, 2021) highlights a digital divide in the uptake of services with 42 per cent of carers welcoming virtual online GP appointments, although 14 per cent found this made their caring role harder (Carers UK, 2021, p. 31). Carers also identified many barriers to digital engagement such as lack of access to IT equipment, a lack of privacy and communication issues for those suffering with dementia or another disability. Many others highlighted the benefits of digital access to services and information, however, so the importance of offering a choice is emphasised as well as taking care not to exclude a significant proportion of the public (*State of Caring*, Carers UK, 2021, p. 33).

In a digital age, we still have to be aware that about a third of people do not want to engage digitally or have the means to engage digitally. We must be careful that we are not creating a 'digital divide' where people who will not be coerced into digital banking or digital bills and the rest become 'digitally disabled' and suffer the same fate that people with other disabilities traditionally have. This can sometimes be referred to as 'digital poverty'. Visit the Digital Poverty Alliance (see Useful websites) to find out more about this topic.

Does digital creativity enhance person-centred care?

Case study: co-creating a digital sexual health clinic in the UK

A UK hospital in the North West approached Chrysalis transsexual support group with a view to co-creating a weekly transsexual health clinic alongside the usual sexual health clinic, arguably the first in the country. This was initially driven by technology, as the nursing staff at the clinic had noticed a discrepancy between statistical instances of trans people with problems and the number of people actually coming forward. Work began before coronavirus reared its head. As the hospital is only an hour away from Chrysalis, everything was done by face-to-face meeting initially. When the pandemic hit, a means had to be found to continue the work remotely. The NHS eventually made Microsoft Teams the standard form of remote communication, and the agility of a digital platform soon showed advantages, not least the capability of holding meetings with distributed people and sharing documentation without printing. Another useful adjunct was the possibility of holding two consecutive meetings 65 miles apart without the aid of a Harrier jump jet! There was still the need to physically trial access systems, but the instances of one-to-one contact became vanishingly small. This case study is a good example of what can be achieved by willing and technologically able people.

Activity 5.4   Critical and creative thinking

Consider how you might address the issue of converting clinic services if they had to return to remote delivery in the future:

- What decisions would you need to take and when?
- What could you do to support people in engaging and feeling comfortable online?
- What else have we learnt in the health and social care sector during the pandemic that could benefit services in the longer term?

An outline answer is provided at the end of this chapter.

The above case study showcases a digital service which enhanced person-centred care through the difficult lockdown period. However, digital engagement can be both a blessing and a curse in that it can create rich, more accessible information systems, but also it exposes the difficulty of connecting people to information who either can't or won't engage digitally. If due regard isn't given to the needs of non-technological people, then this may create a two-tier health system with the technological haves competing unfairly with the technological have nots.

There are times when digital technology can be a barrier to good communication. Within the field of mental health nursing, for instance, we have an immediate need to read body language, as acute mental health issues often cannot easily be communicated verbally and certainly cannot be communicated digitally.

When working with children and young people, it is often the case that their body language will be entirely at odds with what is being said, particularly in cases where there is a safeguarding issue. Not only are there difficulties in reading non-verbal communication, there are also safeguarding issues with not knowing who else may be in the room with the child. This raises the potential for coercion and confidentiality problems.

Service user and carer groups have also raised concerns with medical professionals such as GPs offering a telephone appointment-only policy, with no digital engagement whatsoever. GPs who have engaged digitally have expressed mixed feelings about it, often because of the reasons outlined above, such as confidentiality and barriers to the holistic observation of the signs and symptoms relating to health and well-being.

There is a need to have a 'blended' approach to person-centred care with digital engagement and face-to-face contact playing to their respective strengths, and time taken to 'step back' from the headlong approach of the last 18 months to reconcile, reflect and then build on what has been achieved.

Chapter summary

Our aims at the beginning of this chapter were to encourage you as nurses to consider how to co-create digital content for patients and families to promote person-centred care. We reflected on the shift in the delivery of care from 'doing to you' to 'working with you', which fundamentally impacts on your professional role as a nurse. We hope you enjoyed exploring our examples from practice where we have engaged the views of service users and carers, and co-designed digital resources for education and practice. By unleashing your digital creativity, we hope that you will extend your reach as a care-provider by engaging with more patients and families, while being mindful of the challenges these can bring. The last two years of living through a global pandemic have forced us all to change our ways of communicating and embracing a blended approach of face-to-face and online connectivity will be our collective future.

Activities: brief outline answers

Activity 5.1 Reflection (page 74)

1. The Comensus group of service users and carers were initially reluctant to be filmed sharing their experiences, as they thought this meant that they would no longer be invited into the university to participate in teaching. However, staff worked hard to alleviate these concerns and Comensus members are now reassured that students and learners are able to watch online resources in their own time and still engage with them in the classroom to ask

questions. Online learning has also meant a reduction in travel time and early starts for our service user and carer group.

2. Students and learners have commented that they prefer face-to-face engagement in the main. However, they also see the benefit of being able to view films and other resources at home, in their own time and ask questions later on.

Activity 5.2   Digital co-creativity (page 76)

A digital resource would be a great way of collating images and information about the benefits of walking for well-being and also for signposting people to local groups. You could ask a local patient group if anyone wished to contribute their experiences, while paying particular emphasis on protecting people's anonymity. Your practice surgery or health community hub may already have a web page which you could add to, or some financial support may be available to develop your own.

Activity 5.3   Barriers and enablers to digital creativity (page 79)

The key barriers to co-production are: time, culture, resources, power issues and access. The key enablers are: training and support, time, relationship-building, authenticity, open culture of engagement.

Activity 5.4   Critical and creative thinking (page 82)

A primary consideration is ensuring that service users and carers' details are up to date and include relevant email and telephone information. Special consideration should be given to those who have previously not engaged - how will these people be supported? Is there any funding to support a loan scheme for digital technology to be made available to them? Is there a local community hub that can provide support for this service? During the recent pandemic, we learnt that people relied on regular human connection, even if this was through remote means or via a telephone call. Remember that people always welcome having a choice if possible.

Useful websites

www.gov.uk/service-manual/technology/how-to-test-frontend-performance

UK Government guidance and standards about size of internet pages and speed of access.

www.transsexualinfo.co.uk

The Chrysalis Transexual Support Group's website.

www.uclan.ac.uk/values-and-initiatives/comensus

University of Central Lancashire's Community Engagement and Service User Support group (Comensus).

www.champspublichealth.com/new-lower-my-drinking-campaign-launched-in-cheshire-mersey-side-to-help-with-increased-covid-related-drinking

Champs app: enables service users to manage their own alcohol use and use online tools to reduce harmful levels of use.

https://digitalpovertyalliance.org

The Digital Poverty Alliance: a group leading sustainable action against digital poverty.

Chapter 6

Digital curation: implications for the nursing student and nursing practice

Dilla Davis

HEE Digital Capabilities Framework

This chapter will address the following domains of digital capability:

Communication, collaboration and participation (level 2)

- Demonstrate safer, positive, sensitive and appropriate attitudes and behaviours in relation to online/digital communication, collaboration and participation

Information, data and content (level 2)

- Use digital tools to search and locate accurate, reliable and safe information and content
- Follow the steps required to test the accuracy of information, data and content
- Evaluate digital content to test for bias, misinformation, relevance

Teaching, learning and self-development (level 2)

- Use digital tools and technologies to support personal learning
- Evaluate information to support personal and professional learning

---

Chapter aims

After reading this chapter, you will be able to:

- understand the term 'curation' and the complexity of information curation;
- appreciate the importance of evaluation of curated information in student learning and patient empowerment;
- understand the curation process, the metacognition underlying the process and the tools for evaluating digital content.

Introduction

The proliferation of social web (technologies and platforms) that allows people to engage in the user-generated process has created a massive volume of information by members of the public, yet organisations are still sceptical to utilise it. Questions such as 'Is the information trustworthy, real, valuable, credible?' remain. Another challenge associated with this phenomenon is being able to navigate through the volume of information shared. In this chapter, curation tools (see Figure 6.1) and the curation processes are discussed to equip the reader with knowledge on how to curate. It will explore co-curation with colleagues, patients, families and carers where appropriate.

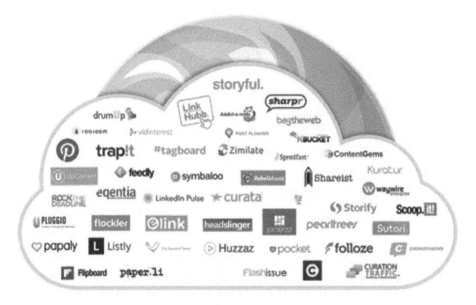

Figure 6.1 Curation tools (adapted from: www.curata.com/blog/content-curation-tools-the-ultimate-list)

Every minute, 571 new websites are launched and 48 hours of video uploaded. Everyday, 175 million tweets are sent (Buck, 2013). In the past, information was reserved for experts and filtered out for the public, but now information is always rapidly accessible and from anywhere. As a result, finding information is no longer difficult. The task lies in sorting through millions of results returned in a single Google search. Finding trustworthy content among the enormous amount of online content is, in fact, one of the major issues we face. There is a need for the skill and ability to distinguish between a variety of unreliable internet resources and those that consistently offer high-quality health and medical information.

The NHS must increase its awareness of ethical issues, develop its data origin, management and governance skills, and hone its critical assessment abilities (Topol, 2019). All healthcare workers should get education and training in the creation, integration and management of health data, the ethics of autonomous systems and tools, and the evaluation and explanation of robotics and artificial intelligence (AI) technology. For autonomous and data-driven technologies to succeed, the workforce must be specially trained in essential skills and have expertise in data management, governance and data origin. NHS personnel must be trained to utilise AI confidently and appropriately since it is a tool, just like any other tool in the healthcare industry. The foundations of AI and machine learning are founded on digital management, statistics and probability, and today's NHS personnel will need to be proficient in these fields to be proficient users of these tools of the future.

Moreover, lessons and textbooks are no longer the only ways that students learn. Instead, they are looking for free knowledge online to supplement what they are learning through textbooks and lectures. Students will also need to gain knowledge in health data provenance, curation, integration and governance because it will be routinely used to gather information about patients' wellness, and not just for the care of individual patients, but also for the well-being of the entire population.

What is curation?

A curator is defined as one who has the care and superintendence of something, especially one in charge of a museum, zoo or other place of exhibit (*Merriam-Webster Online Dictionary*, 2014) and a curator *gathers, evaluates, and contextualises web information and content of a specific sort into a platform or into an understandable manner* (Buck, 2013). In other words, content curation is the process of analysing, classifying, organising web content around a certain theme (*Macmillan Dictionary*, 2014). The ability to seek, gather and filter content using technology is crucial, as is the capacity to contextualise and assess content and to produce evaluative summaries and standardised ratings. Moreover, curation is the act of giving current content new context by applying fresh viewpoints (Minocha and Petre, 2012).

The use of digital curation can improve education in a variety of ways. Because of the levelling ability of the new curation tools, networks for professional learning are enabled to create and hone their own interests and collections of materials in startlingly simple, efficient and timely ways (Navarro et al., 2021). The 'participatory' cultural context of digital curation (Jenkins et al., 2009) makes it possible for regular people to annotate, appropriate, archive and recirculate digital content through the use of technology. Rather than serve the pervasive hegemony, these average users have the capacity to wrestle power and authority from the traditional established estates of media, government and academia, and construct new or frame existing articulations/paradigms of knowledge to serve their own needs. Such powerful acquisition and ownership lead to innovative modes of engagement, enabling a platform for critical reappraisal, and for interrogating reflection and scrutiny at both personal and community levels (Flintoff et al., 2014).

> ## Activity 6.1   Reflection
>
> Reflect on the factors that would influence you if you were building content for Generation Z. Now read the blog https://socialnomics.net/2019/05/09/how-to-shape-your-content-for-generation-z-consumers/
>
> - What concepts would you reflect on while curating content for Generation Z?
> - Did you think about these concepts prior to reading the blog?
> - Do you agree with these concepts?
>
> *An outline answer is provided at the end of this chapter.*

Why should we evaluate information?

Since the advent of the internet, anyone can publish material online for a variety of purposes. The usage of online information (digital content), including blogs, wikis, websites and social media, can result in the dissemination of inaccurate information that is factually and medically erroneous. In order to provide patients with the best care possible, it is crucial to identify the information that is accurate, trustworthy and clear among the large array of information that is readily available. Digital literacy is about being able to identify high-quality, trustworthy and evidence-based digital content.

Evaluating information is an essential part of digital literacy and it is crucial to teach pupils of all ages and academic levels this digital literacy skill. In fact, traditional types of courses where information is delivered more didactically and systematically by faculty – a structure adopted by textbooks – required less searching for information by students (Cole et al., 2017). Since the curriculum has changed, students are now required to do information searches in order to understand the case they are studying and to take responsibility for their own learning. Multimedia resources can be accessible at a time and location that is convenient for the student. When looking for an answer to a particular question, many individuals turn to the internet first due to its accessibility and the simplicity of search engines like Google. However, individuals might use unreliable or low-quality internet sources and rely too much on Wikipedia rather than sources that have undergone peer review, which is a worry that is reflected in the literature.

There are a tonne of resources for information, including more than 40,000 education apps, innumerable YouTube videos, audio lectures and tutorials on undertaking a patient's health history, listening to their heartbeat or changing a sterile dressing. The content that students will use in their regular contacts with clients, patients, service users and their families and communities is another kind to curate. A nursing student requires assistance selecting the 'best' app to use to instruct a patient or make a client recommendation, vetting this type of content for clinical relevance and appropriateness. This includes apps that inform users about ailments and different types of medications, or apps that let users monitor their vital signs, blood sugar levels or diet. The foundation of patient care is determining whether content is clinically acceptable and relevant.

To ascertain whether digital content is meaningful, one needs to:

- look at the information critically to determine its applicability, suitability and reliability;
- scrutinise the sources of information for authenticity;
- verify that information and resources are fit for purpose; and
- check for currency, accuracy and validity, as these serve as indicators of information quality.

Critical evaluation of information involves assessing the authorship, the reliability and authenticity of the information at hand. This paradigm is based on the fundamental concepts of meta literacy, with a particular emphasis on metacognition, or critical self-reflection, as being essential for increasing one's level of self-direction in the fast-evolving digital ecosystem.

The meta literacy framework

Cognitive and metacognitive skills alongside managing tools and disseminating content skills are essential for content curation (Dale, 2014). Meta literacy is a broad range of skills that students must possess in order to be successful participants in collaborative settings as information consumers and creators.

Meta literacy entails:

- understanding the format type and delivery method;
- analysing user comments and feedback as an active researcher;
- establishing a context for user-generated data and critically assessing dynamic content;
- creating original content in multiple media formats;
- understanding issues related to intellectual property, personal privacy, information ethics;
- information exchange in collaborative settings.

(Mackey and Jacobson, 2011)

Content curation promotes digital skills, critical thinking sharing and exchange of knowledge, collaborative learning and personalised learning (Ostashewski et al., 2014). From Reig's (2010) perspective, a content curator is a critical intermediary of knowledge, someone who continuously searches, groups and shares what is most relevant in their field of specialisation. Content curation represents an evolution in information management activity in such a way that the person who carries out this activity becomes a critical knowledge broker (Guallar, 2021). The work of such knowledge brokers or learners is anchored in the six frames of information meta literacy, of which four frames are shown in Figure 6.2.

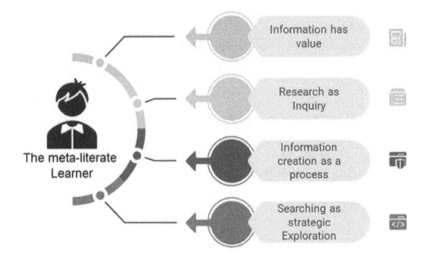

Figure 6.2 Frames of information meta literacy (adapted from ACRL (2015), available at: www.ala.org/acrl/sites/ala.org.acrl/files/content/issues/infolit/framework1.pdf)

- **Information creation as a process**
  Information in any format is produced to convey a message and shared via a selected delivery method. This iterative process of researching, creating, revising and disseminating information varies and the resulting product reflects these differences.

- **Information has value**
  Information possesses several dimensions of value, including as a commodity, as a means of education, as a means of influence and as a means of negotiating and understanding the world.

- **Research as enquiry**
  Research is iterative and depends upon asking increasingly complex questions or new questions whose answers in turn develop additional questions or lines of enquiry in any field.

- **Searching as strategic exploration**
  Information is often linear and iterative, requiring the evaluation of a range of information sources and the mental flexibility to pursue alternate avenues as new understanding develops.

Meta literacy necessitates behavioural (use of tools and techniques), affective, cognitive and metacognitive interaction with the information ecosystem.

The tools for evaluating digital content

Particularly in an internet setting, not all information is reliable. A variety of tools are available that are often used to evaluate digital content. Below are some examples (and there will be an exploration of the CRAAP test in more detail).

- The 5 Ws of website evaluation – Who, What, When, Where and Why.
- Applying the CRAAP (Currency, Relevance, Authority, Accuracy, Purpose) tool.
- RADCAB (Relevance, Appropriateness, Detail, Currency, Authority, Bias) for information evaluation.
- Evaluate it: a guide from Community College of Baltimore library in the USA.
- Evaluating sources: a comprehensive guide from Berkeley University in California for both print and digital resources.
- Truth, Truthiness and Triangulation: news literacy toolkit for the Post Truth world.

The CRAAP Test was created by librarians at California State University, Chico, and is a useful checklist to use when assessing any resource, including web resources (Fielding, 2019). As was already indicated, there are other approaches that might be better suitable, but since the CRAAP tool was one of the first to evaluate online content, it is the subject of this chapter.

The CRAAP tool/test

When determining if a source is trustworthy and reputable enough to employ, the test presents a set of questions to ask oneself.

Currency: consider whether the information's publication date is appropriate for your project.

- What is the publication, copyright or posting date?
- Why does the date matter or not matter for the source's message or content?
- Is the material still relevant to the subject?

Relevance: evaluate the information's suitability for your project.

- For what demographic or educational level (general, experts/scholars) is the information written for?
- Explain why you would or would not quote/reference the information from this source in your project.

Authority: determine if the source author, creator or publisher of the information is the most knowledgeable.

- Who is the author, creator or publisher of the source, or what organisation is responsible for the source?
- Is the contact information readily available?
- How do you know if the author is an expert on the topic – e.g., examine the author's credentials, experience and/or organisational affiliation?
- What is the source of funding?

Accuracy: evaluate the content's dependability, veracity and correctness.

- Is the content well researched or does it have enough support, or neither?
- What kind of language, metaphors and/or tone is employed – e.g., passionate, impartial, etc.?
- Do the premises, claims and conclusions have supporting evidence?
- Are statements made about the truth supported by evidence/cited in the text, in notes or in a bibliography?

Purpose: determine the background of the information's existence.

- Why was this material published – for example, to inform, teach, amuse, persuade?
- How might the author's affiliation affect the point of view, slant or potential bias of the source?
- What conclusions are presented and is the information complete?
- Is anything major excluded?
- How does this resource compare to others on the same topic?

Evaluating information only forms part of the content creation or curation. Several steps/phases are mentioned in literature. Below are examples.

Steps in curating information

Dr Jon Landis, writing about the profound and permanent shift in content access, proposed three steps for content creation (Brooks, 2014): 1) truth vetting – fact checking, examining evidence-based information; 2) critiquing it in terms of its quality and accuracy; and 3) meaning making – interpreting and using this information correctly.

Valenza et al. (2014) offers a snapshot of digital curation practice, revealing how the survey participants (library professionals) define and engage in social media curation (Figure 6.3).

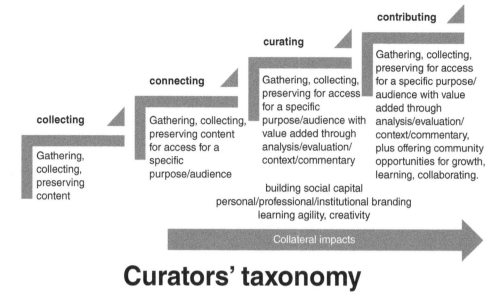

Curators' taxonomy

Figure 6.3 A taxonomy of digital curation (adapted from Valenza et al., 2014; © Copyright 1996–2019, American Library Association)

Guallar (2020) defines the methodology of content curation in four steps, called the '4Ss model': search, select, sense making and share (see Figure 6.4).

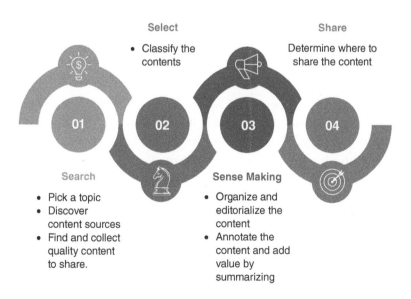

Figure 6.4 Four steps in curation (Guallar, 2020)

Case study: Sky

Sky is a first-year nursing student. During class, her group was tasked with going away and curating a list of relevant scientific articles around the cardiovascular system.

After reading the chapter on curation in this book, Sky was able to lead her group on the project.

Activity 6.2   Reflection

Reflect on the information that enabled Sky to lead her group. What skills might you need to develop to become a good curator?

An outline answer is provided at the end of this chapter.

Characteristics of a good curator

A good curator knows how to find, aggregate and synthesise reliable information, putting it into context for their communities and sharing it in a format that is easy to access and understand.

Consider the source The most crucial first step in selecting reliable information is this one. Use the NHS trust/university library search facility as the first point and then the databases. Curate information exclusively from trustworthy and reputable sources.

Set the scene/provide the context The fundamental components of content curation include being able to condense the main ideas, providing your own perspective and placing things in a context that makes sense to your community. It is not about gathering links or being an information hoarder. What have experts in the field discovered? What are the latest recommendations for medical care? Or how have other patients dealt with what I'm describing?

Use the correct tools Wikis, Facebook, Pinterest and Wakelet have all been used successfully in a variety of learning and teaching applications, including creating and curating resources on nursing informatics, acting as an interactive online final year project notebook and fostering professionalism in medical students. The platforms can all facilitate group learning and they might aid in the growth of digital literacy, critical thinking abilities and knowledge of broader health issues in society. Readers can leave comments on curators' posts, fostering a collaborative environment. Wakelet, for example, is a tool that is helpful for organising and archiving. But for these tools to be used to their full potential, staff and students must receive enough training, have a chance to experience utilising them and receive continuing support.

Develop the ability to read beyond headlines It is critical to understand how to separate fact from fiction. If the news story provides evidence to back up its claims, keep reading to discover the study's most significant findings. Seek out the article's expert feedback from doctors or other knowledgeable healthcare commentators.

Reference Always cite the original source when curating content.

Register for alerts and newsletters Create Google alerts for the healthcare subjects that are relevant to your community. Include Google Scholar, which indexes the majority of European and American peer-reviewed online publications.

Use social media to its full potential Share your curated content via your social networks and make it easy for others to share it too.

A good curator makes use of the appropriate curating tool and curating technique. The following passages provide an outline for these tools and techniques.

Curating tools

Anyone can now create and curate content thanks to digital tools, which also make it possible for someone with a narrowly concentrated interest to identify and gather online artefacts to share with their intended audience. An additional layer of quality control is added by curators. They can remove a lot of the unimportant content, allowing the best content to rise to the top. The end user can quickly and simply add objects to their own collections as well as further filter and improve the collection using many of the new digital creation tools. More than just copying and pasting links into a Word document is involved in creating an online collection of information. The abundance of internet curation tools makes it possible for nurses to develop straightforward platforms that can be utilised with students to assemble and arrange their online research or to generate a list of pertinent films for a particular teaching topic. When utilised appropriately, curation technologies and techniques can eliminate the need for writing by simplifying, organising and sharing these internet resources.

Curating techniques

There are many techniques available for curating content and here are some examples:

• **Natural language processing** Computer science, artificial intelligence and linguistics all have fields called 'natural language processing' that study how computers and human (natural) languages interact. In more detail, it is the procedure through which a computer generates natural language output or extracts relevant information from natural language input – for example, Alexa.

- **News analytics** The measuring of the many qualitative and quantitative characteristics of textual (unstructured data) news items is known as 'news analytics'. Sentiment, relevancy and novelty are a few of the characteristics analysed.
- **Opinion mining** Opinion mining (sentiment mining, opinion/sentiment extraction) aims to create automatic systems that can extract human opinions from natural language text.
- **Scraping** These are all terms used to describe the process of gathering unstructured text data from social media and other websites.
- **Sentiment analysis** The technique of identifying and extracting subjective information from source materials using text analytics, computational linguistics and natural language processing.
- **Text analytics** This involves information retrieval – for example, lexical analysis is the study of word frequency distributions, pattern recognition, tagging/annotation, information extraction, data-mining techniques, including link and association analysis, visualisation and predictive analytics.

Curating tools

Digital curation tools have allowed anyone to become a creator and a curator, allowing a person with a focused interest in a specific topic to find and collect artefacts on the internet to share with their target audience. Curators add a level of quality control around a topic. They can filter a lot of the less important content and allow quality material to surface to the top. Many of the new digital creation tools allow for the end user to further filter and refine the collection, and to quickly and easily add items to their own collection. Creating an online curation of resources goes far beyond the simple copying and pasting of links to a Word document. The vast amount of curation tools online allows nurses to create simple platforms and can also be used with students who need to compile and organise their online research or use it to aggregate a list of applicable videos for a specific teaching topic. Curation tools and curating skills, when used properly, can help to simplify, organise and share these online resources without picking up a pen. Moreover, it can lead to patient empowerment.

Patient empowerment and nurse curation skills

Facebook and YouTube are the social networks that are most regularly used by people of all ages to get health information, while more recent research has also noted the significant use of WhatsApp as a source for finding and accessing health information (Marar et al., 2019). The topics they consult are very diverse, although they tend to mostly focus on information about different life stages like pregnancy or menopause, the management of chronic diseases like diabetes or hypertension or the use of medication (Zucco et al., 2018). Patients may have adequate digital skills and have the ability to consult health information on the internet, but this does not imply that it is correctly understood (Kobayashi and Ishizaki, 2019) or may give erroneous results (Marcu et al., 2019).

Many users view health content on YouTube. However, this content may be erroneous or confusing and may not provide quality information (Cassidy et al., 2018; Jain et al., 2019). The quality of healthcare professional and patient encounter is lessened when this information is not confirmed with a nurse or doctor, or when they do not show any interest in the information obtained by the patient (Wong and Cheung, 2019). As it can be frustrating for the patient to find contradictory information and not be able to discuss it, it is essential that the nurse is able to guide the patient in the search for quality information in order to reduce anxiety and minimise inadequate encounters or consultations. Such endorsements or validations can strengthen the professional–patient relationship (Tan and Goonawardene, 2017). However, the main barrier pointed out by nurses when it comes to consulting and confirming valid information on the internet is a lack of time, followed by a lack of skills in this area (Khodaveisi, 2020).

Co-curating with the patient for chronic illness management

Nurses check and monitor that patients acquire the skills they need for self-care and self- management of their health. Nevertheless, few digital resources have been offered or created by nurses for patients, even though they are effective methods of monitoring the chronically ill (Madrigal and Escoffery, 2018). The best way to develop quality resources is in partnership with the patient as an adviser and guide (Featherall, 2018).

Activity 6.3   Evaluating information credibility

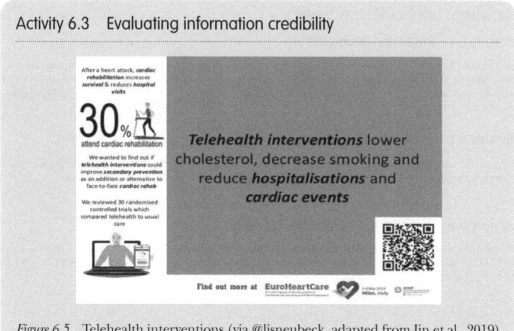

Figure 6.5   Telehealth interventions (via @lisneubeck, adapted from Jin et al., 2019)

(Continued)

(Continued)

The image above is taken from a tweet. Look at the information provided. Reflect on whether you would probe further. Use the CRAAP tool to evaluate and ascertain if the information is credible and reliable, and whether it will pass the CRAAP test.

http://library.truman.edu/library_instruction/craaptestworksheet.pdf

An outline answer is provided at the end of this chapter.

Chapter summary

Just as there are curators for art galleries, nurses need to be curators for their professional practice. Curation is the process of gathering information from various sources that is pertinent to your patients, organising it for your own use and then thoughtfully disseminating it to other nurses. Curating internet information not only enables you to identify resources beneficial to your particular need, but it also enables you to give back by assisting other nurses who are conducting comparable searches to locate those resources. By doing this, you establish an online community that welcomes explorers looking for original, interesting and practical methods.

Activities: brief outline answers

Activity 6.1   Reflection (page 88)

You should be able to reflect on the quick tips: explore interactive content; work/collaborate with influencers; focus on quality, not quantity; short-form content does better; be genuine, be yourself; be accountable and lend support to social causes; don't lump in Gen-Z with the millennials.

Activity 6.2   Reflection (page 94)

Sky could use the four-step model to outline the project – delegate the responsibilities and through constructive discussions determine how and where to share the information.

Activity 6.3   Evaluating information credibility (page 97)

It will pass the CRAAP test. The clues on the tweet information are Randomised Control Trial, ESC (European Cardiology Society) etc. and should prompt the reader to probe deeper – to go to the primary source.

Chapter 7 · Digital innovation in healthcare

Yeliz Prior and Matthew Wynn

HEE Digital Capabilities Framework

This chapter will address the following domains of digital capability:

Creation, innovation and research (level 2)

- Innovative use of digital technologies to support healthcare and new innovative ways of working and thinking
- Access, analyse, interpret and evaluate evidence appropriate for specific research and/or scholarship activities

Digital identity, wellbeing, safety and security (level 2)

- The ability to demonstrate and champion ethical, positive, healthy and appropriate attitudes and behaviours

Information, data and content literacies (level 2)

- Abide by legislation, guidelines, policies and protocols to protect privacy, copyright and intellectual property in the use and sharing of digital media, information and data

Chapter aims

After reading this chapter, you will be able to:

- explore the process and impact of digital innovation in healthcare;
- identify methodological approaches to digital health research;
- understand the core ethical principles for digital health innovation and research;
- consider the implications of data regulations for digital health research.

Introduction

Healthcare systems are continuously evolving to meet rising challenges such as the growing and ageing population, evolving healthcare needs due to the increase in cases of obesity, long-term conditions, dementia, mental health issues and antibiotic resistance. This burden was further stress-tested by the coronavirus (COVID-19) pandemic, which placed unprecedented demands on the health service systems, capacity and capability to continue to deliver care to the expected standards. Nevertheless, this growing pressure has led to medical care advancements and technological innovations at a pace and scale that was unimaginable prior to the pandemic. In 2020, the first national Chief Nursing Information Officer for England was appointed to lead nursing and midwifery strategy in the safe and effective care of their patients through use of technology. This led to a publication of a White Paper to outline the renewed commitment to ensuring more effective data sharing across the health and care system, and digital transformation of care pathways (DoH, 2022).

The era of digital innovations in healthcare includes a wide range of technologies, such as applications (apps), programs and software used in the healthcare system and the public domain. These innovations have a great potential to support healthcare delivery via strategic data management to enable coordinated care across multidisciplinary teams and involve patients to take a more active role in their treatment towards individualised care. These technologies may be stand-alone or combined with other products such as medical devices or diagnostic tests (NICE, 2022) and have the capacity to transform both the mode and quality of healthcare by digitising nursing informatics (computational systems for data storage and retrieval), reduce time spent on documentation, release time for care, improve safety and reduce avoidable harm, strengthen evidence base for nursing interventions, and empower people to actively participate and contribute to their care (NHS England, 2021).

Digital innovations in healthcare

Technology has long been associated with the delivery of healthcare. From ancient healers using primitive surgical tools to perform ill-advised lobotomies to modern-day smart watches capable of monitoring heart rhythms and blood oxygen saturation, technology has always featured in the practice of care. Digital innovations, however, have altered the ways in which both professionals and patients interact with technology and data, ultimately impacting both decision making and clinical outcomes. In a study by Iyawa et al. (2016), 11 different components and sources of innovation were described. These include the influences of product developers, users and sociopolitical factors associated with the process of technological development.

The adoption of those best-demonstrated practices that have been proven to be successful and implementation of those practices aimed at improving treatment, diagnosis, education, outreach, prevention and research, and with the long term goals of improving quality, safety, outcomes, efficiency and costs.

(Iyawa et al., 2016)

The paradigm shift towards digital approaches to healthcare has been suggested to potentially lead to a 'democratisation' of care in the long term, ultimately creating an equal professional–patient relationship within which both parties have equal access to information and data related to the care they give/receive (Mesko et al., 2017).

Understanding the history of digital innovations and the research evidence indicating their impact can help us to appreciate both their current and potential future value. In Figure 7.1 below you can see a timeline highlighting the introduction of significant new digital technologies and developments of online information sources which have impacted healthcare over the last 150 years.

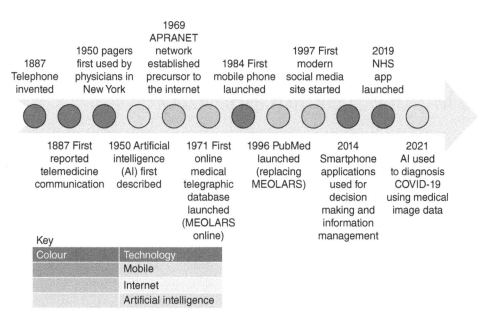

Figure 7.1   Key milestones in digital technology innovation and development for healthcare

As can be seen from the timeline below (Figure 7.2), digital innovation over the last 15 years has been rapid and has had a profound impact on ways that health professionals interact with patients and information. It highlights the near-exponential increase in the number of articles indexed in PubMed using the keywords 'digital innovation'.

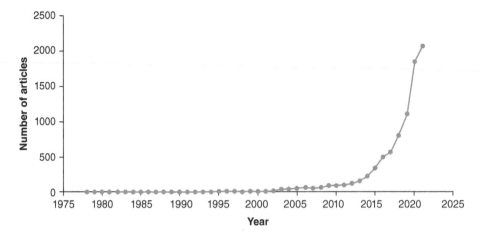

Figure 7.2 Articles including the term 'digital innovation' indexed in PubMed over time (PubMed, 2022)

The chart shows that more articles were published about digital innovation in healthcare in 2021 than in the years 1978–2015 combined. It is therefore not unreasonable to assume that the rate of digital innovation will continue into the future given the recent explosion of interest in this area of study. Critically, nurses must consider what the potential impacts of this innovation might be.

The impact of digital innovations

To explore the potential impacts of digital innovations on nursing practice, we will consider digital innovation in a key area of nursing practice and explore the research evidence indicating its impact. In the following research summary, we will consider the potential impact of electronic medication systems (EMS) on the processes involved in medicines administration.

Research summary: medicine administration

The administration of medicines is an important part of many nurses' roles. Correct administration can improve patients' health and save lives. However, if errors are made, the impacts can be potentially fatal for patients. Nurses are typically taught that they must consider the 'nine rights' of medicine administration, which are right patient, right medicine, right route, right time, right dose, right documentation, right action, right form and right response in order to avoid drug errors (Elliot and Liu, 2013). Perhaps because of the significant safety risks inherent in medicines administration, digital solutions for improving safety during this process have been investigated by researchers. These digital technologies aim to prevent drug errors through a combination of alerts, prompts and remote communication between professionals.

EMS are now available which can perform or assist with the following processes related to medicines administration:

- Prescribing
- Dispensing
- Pharmacy referrals

(Goundrey-Smith, 2019)

A recent review on the effectiveness of EMS for improving the safety of medicines administration highlighted the potential benefits to these systems (Gates et al., 2020). The authors reported that use of EMS is associated with significantly reduced rates of medication errors. However, the authors also reported that there is still insufficient evidence indicating how effective these systems are for preventing serious harm to patients. Notably, an earlier study by Davies et al. (2017) investigating the impact of electronic prescribing systems on staff perceptions of safety in an English hospital reported a reduction in perceived safety when using electronic prescribing systems. The authors concluded that poor implementation strategies and poor staff competence may have been responsible for the poor perceptions of the technology. It is clear that EMS has the potential to prevent medication errors when used correctly. However, without staff having the appropriate digital skills and a well-considered implementation plan, the benefits of this technology may be diminished.

The research summary highlights that the implementation of digital innovations in nursing practice has the potential to improve the safety of practice. However, careful attention must be given to how new technologies are implemented. Specifically, if staff do not feel they have sufficient skills to utilise technology, this may damage perceptions of its value and consequently limit its value or uptake in practice. As a nurse, it is important to ensure that relevant skills are kept up to date and, where necessary, new skills are developed to ensure we can translate the implementation of new technology into improved clinical outcomes for patients. Finally, it is evident that in the case of EMS, more evidence is required to fully elucidate its impact on harms experienced by patients. With the recent rapid increase in digital innovation, it may be the case that not all technologies have been robustly evaluated. Nurses must be mindful of this fact and ensure that over-dependence on digital solutions does not come at the cost of sound clinical judgement and reasoning.

Unintended consequences of digital innovation

While there is great potential for digital innovation to improve the care that patients receive, it has already been associated with a number of negative unintended consequences. A study by Ziebland et al. (2021) investigated these potential consequences and reported three broad themes in their manifestations. First, the use of digital tools may cause disrupted power relations between patients and professionals, and between professionals. Notably, in cases where e-messaging processes were used, doctors felt they had less power to exercise their own judgement over whether their input was required clinically when requests from nurses were automatically recorded in digital records. Where remote consultations were offered, an increase in clinicians yielding to patients' requests was observed – e.g., for prescriptions or visitation (Mehrotra et al., 2013). This was attributed to the ability for patients to 'shop around' for alternative digital health consultations, making clinicians feel less able to reject patient requests. Second, paradoxical outcomes may be noted such as 'e-iatrogenesis'. This has been defined as *patient harm caused at least in part by the application of health information technology* (Weiner et al., 2007). Digital innovations are intended to improve not worsen clinical outcomes, making this a worrying finding. Harms reported may be due to omission or commission. Examples may include incorrect prescribing (commission) in a digital record, or cases of clinicians copying and pasting digital notes rather than updating them, leading to omission of important information. The final theme reported by Ziebland et al. (2021) was the establishment of potentially unhelpful cultures affecting both patients and clinicians. For example, clinicians reported the feeling of being watched by management staff in some cases where digital processes were utilised. Patients were reported to contribute to a culture of 'gaming' systems where digital technology was used to administer clinic appointments – for example, by providing details on booking systems to ensure a face-to-face appointment was offered when it was not required. It is also important to consider the impact of digital innovation on health inequalities. The COVID-19 pandemic highlighted the stark differences in the level of access to healthcare provided using internet or digital communication based technologies (van Laar, 2020). Individuals who are less educated, elderly and have low literacy skills have been identified as the most likely to miss out on opportunities for improved health provided by digital technologies (Office for National Statistics, 2021).

Nurses must be vigilant to these potential sources of digital harm and mitigate them where possible. The impacts of digital innovation that were not intended may nonetheless be anticipated. Nurses must reflect on their use of digital technologies and consider how issues like e-iatrogenesis may occur and make efforts to prevent it.

Digital sources of information

Throughout history, individuals responsible for the care of the diseased or wounded have required sources of information to support their approach to care. Perhaps one of the earliest and most famous examples is the Edwin Smith papyrus, a 22-page scroll which is thought to be nearly 3,000 years old. This document contained within it practical guidance on how to treat wounds based on the experience of its author. It even detailed which types of wounds had a known treatment, which had uncertain treatments, and which had none at all (Brawanski, 2021). These early attempts to document and store information presented issues to people delivering healthcare at the time. For example, you had to be able to access the scroll (or any other documentation medium) to know its contents and heed its guidance. There was no robust system for keeping the information contained within it up to date and there was little certainty that the information contained within it could be relied upon.

Fast forward over 2,000 years to 1984 and the first online bibliographic database of nursing literature went online – the Cumulative Index to Nursing and Allied Health Literature (CINAHL). Bibliographic databases provide an index of journal articles from many different journals. This addresses issues of the past by making robust, peer-reviewed evidence available digitally without you having to travel to the nearest medical scroll repository. Fast forward again, however, and you find a proliferation of low-quality information sources, providing unreliable information related to healthcare. It was observed during the COVID-19 pandemic that this can lead to an 'infodemic', defined by the World Health Organization (2021) as *too much information including false or misleading information in digital and physical environments during a disease outbreak*. This information is often shared via social media platforms such as Facebook, Twitter and Reddit, and may have negative impacts on clinical outcomes and relationships between patients and healthcare professionals (Suarez-Lledo and Alvarez-Galvez, 2021).

This highlights the importance of understanding where reliable information can be found. In the information age, we have progressed from issues related to accessing medical information to issues with being able to access too much information. We must be capable of finding reliable digital sources of information and knowing how to ensure that it is reliable.

It is important to remember that while utilising digital sources of information potentially increases the risk of accessing unreliable information, there are many benefits to digital information sources. First, they can be updated regularly and easily to reflect new evidence. This cannot be done easily with hard documents due to the time taken for the publication process. Second, they can be shared easily – for example, between departments in a hospital, via email or a local intranet. Finally, it is often easier to access than non-digital information due to the widespread ownership of mobile smartphones and access to the internet. Further details on the assessment of information credibility is covered in Chapter 6.

Consider the following scenario and complete the activity.

Scenario: clinical decision making

You are a newly qualified nurse on a general medical ward. A nurse from the emergency department (ED) arrives on the ward to hand over a patient to you. This patient, Miss Jennings, has a grade IV pressure injury on her sacrum which requires a dressing change. The ED nurse hands over that she does not know much about dressings as they are rarely changed in the ED. You ask your colleague for some guidance, but they are unsure as they have only recently started working on the ward after working for several years in an ophthalmology clinic. You note that there are some textbooks in the staffroom, but these are all over ten years old. There is a printed copy of the trust policy on pressure ulcer prevention, but you note that this is also out of date by a number of years.

Activity 7.1   Reflection

Reflect on the scenario above using the following questions:

- What would you do in this situation?
- How and where would you obtain the necessary information?
- Try to access the information you would need in this scenario and write down how you would approach this case.

An outline answer is provided at the end of this chapter.

Digital approaches to health research

As digital health is becoming a large part of healthcare delivery systems, digital approaches to undertake health research is also a rapidly growing and evolving field for novel methodologies. There is an increasing convergence between health informatics, medical technologies and information and communication technology designed for health professionals and patients' use to offer personalised medicine, prediction and prevention of health outcomes to inform clinical diagnosis, treatment, participatory health and research. Moreover, guidelines to inform the development and evaluation of these technologies encourage the involvement and engagement of service users in design to ensure these are fit for purpose to meet the specific needs of system users (Jandoo, 2020; NICE, 2022). As a result, there is a new paradigm in healthcare research towards a participatory model of innovation, called the Maker Movement, promising to lead to novel and transformative solutions for healthcare (Awori and Lee, 2017).

Methodological consideration and challenges

When considering the creation of novel digital approaches to health research methods, data collection, storage, management and analysis can largely differ from the traditional mediums that have been used and tested to date, but the fundamental principle and values behind a good quality, robust research evidence remains unchanged. As the evidence base behind digital approaches to health research is still in its infancy, we know that more research is needed to support the research methods used, and, where possible, digital health research should proceed along conventional lines to follow established protocols for the conduct of clinical trials, controlled case studies and cohort studies (Guo et al., 2020; Kumar et al., 2021; Nebeker et al., 2019).

In the main, challenges to develop robust research protocols for digital approaches to health research stem from the management of large and complex data (e.g., big data) and digital capabilities required to analyse these. Thus, whether you are a health researcher with high digital literacy or not, it is important to start your digital health project with clear aims and objectives, and the rationale behind the research question by considering ways in which you want to advance knowledge and practice in your clinical practice (Gray and Sockolow, 2016). Next, you would need to search the literature to establish any published studies that utilised such systems to collect and analyse health data to get an overview of common models of practice and research protocols followed in similar fields. You would also need to develop a thorough knowledge and understanding of the information communication technology (ICT) systems you are planning to utilise, to include data governance, security, national and organisational guidelines and policies that cover these, as well as the ethical issues related to electronic health records.

If your research project aims to develop a novel technology – e.g., a new clinical tool, outcome measure or platform to support patients or clinicians – it is ultimately your role as a responsible health researcher to ensure that your product is compliant with overarching guidelines and standards, and can support rigorous and transparent research. This may also require the involvement and engagement of advisory services from professional and/or patient organisations, where this new tool will be implemented.

Ethics and eResearch

eResearch in the context of health research refers to the use of ICTs to enable existing and new forms of research sampling, recruitment, data collection, storage, analyses, visualisation and data sharing with human participants. A diverse range of eResearch methods are now evident in health research with:

- internet/online participant recruitment;
- smartphone data collection and interventions;
- internet-based survey and interview;
- digital methods – e.g., data collection from social media (e.g., Twitter feeds, online chat rooms, netrography);
- analysis of the data collected in health settings via electronic medical management databases (e.g., EMS, ePROMs);
- digital photo/video methods;
- ICT-enabled data linkage.

Importantly, eResearch methods are now allowing access to research tools with participants from vulnerable populations (e.g., people with rare diseases, psychopathic traits and deviant sexual interests, youth mental health and drug research) as there are high rates of ICT ownership and utilisation among these groups which are difficult to identify, recruit and retain in research, treatment and prevention programs due to patterns in hidden behaviours and cultural stigmatisation. eResearch methods have additional and proven benefits in both therapeutic (e.g., prevention, treatment and other interventions) and non-therapeutic research (e.g., epidemiological, social and behavioural, humanities) as they are linked with efficiency in treatment delivery, improved treatment protocol monitoring and adherence, increased participant comfort, anonymity and control, as well as reduced research costs and data errors. The benefits of eHealth and eResearch also poses new ethical challenges, as the methodological approaches are developed faster than the guidelines to ensure ethics guidelines to safeguard participants. The use of eHealth services and participation in eResearch should not prejudice the duty of care the clinicians have for participants. Therefore, eHealth data architects and healthcare professionals need to act to maintain and improve user access and data accuracy, and provide different levels of security in eHealth and eResearch relative to the information collected and stored.

Core ethical principles

The code of ethics is built upon a set of principles to guide decision making to promote fair dealings and protect the vulnerable. These standards align with the aims of research, help ensure researchers can be held accountable to the public and engender public support for research (Resnik, 2015). *The Belmont Report* (1979), created following the National Research Act (1974), identifies basic ethical principles and guidelines that address ethical issues arising from the conduct of research with humans. There are seven main principles identified in this report: respect for autonomy and protecting those with diminished autonomy; beneficence and non-maleficence; justice; informed consent; confidentiality and data protection; integrity and conflict of interest. These principles were later adapted by the Association of Medical Research Charities (AMRC) to provide a framework for understanding ethical principles for digital health (AMRC, 2020). These principles are outlined in Table 7.1.

1	Beneficence	Do work that is to the benefit, not detriment of people. The benefits of the work should outweigh the potential risks.
2	Non-maleficence	Avoid harm.
3	Autonomy	Enable people to make choices. This requires people to have sufficient knowledge and understanding to decide.
4	Justice	The benefits and risks should be distributed fairly.
5	Explicability	Transparency around how and why digital health solutions generate the outcomes they do.
6	Sustainability	Minimise risk of developing digital products and services which users become dependent on but cannot be sustained.
7	Open research	Commitment to make research freely open and accessible for reuse.
8	Community mindedness	Willingness to collaborate within the digital health community, such as sharing platforms applicable across medical conditions.
9	Proportionality	Being proportionate to the relevant risk and potential benefit.

Table 7.1 Navigating the digital health ethics landscape (adapted from *Navigating the Digital Health Ethics Landscape: A Framework for Understanding Ethical Principles for Digital Health* © AMRC) (www.amrc.org.uk)

Ethical challenges in eResearch arise from the intersection of new, rapidly evolving technologies; the growing number of stakeholders; big data; novel computational and analytic techniques; and a lack of regulatory controls or common standards to guide this convergence in the health ecosystem (Nebeker et al., 2019). Key considerations such as trust, privacy, data protection, ownership, dignity, and equity and proportionality of response should be well-thought-out prior to the implementation of such technologies to avoid harm. Digital health research must be transparent in such a way that participants need to be reassured that data is being processed properly, that it is up-to-date and of quality, and that security risks are being taken into account to instil trust (EHTEL, 2012). Association of Internet Researchers (AOIR) has also produced a 2002 report to assist researchers in making decisions about internet research, which was updated in 2012, with recommendations from the AoIR Ethics Working Committee (AIOR, 2020). This could be used as a helpful guide to help researchers in making ethical decisions in their research.

Data regulations in the UK

In the UK, the use of personal data is regulated primarily by the GDPR and DPA, and laws on confidentiality vary between different parts of the UK (England, Northern Ireland, Scotland and Wales). The Medicines and Healthcare Product Regulatory (MHRA) is the competent regulatory authority for medical devices and maintains the register for such devices. In addition, various regulatory bodies have responsibility for UK CE/UKCA marking regulations. Key considerations for digital health, eHealth technologies and eResearch are data protection, and especially the lawful transmission, storing processing and use of data, and ensuring that adequate informed consent to such use has been obtained. The providers must ensure that advice and services provided on the platform are fit for purpose, and failure to process information resulting in personal injury may result in liability. Formal endorsement by reputable bodies – e.g., Health Research Authority – further drives the clinical adoption of eHealth technologies (Department of Health and Social Care, 2021).

Case study: Mr Harif

Staff Nurse Susan is a research nurse who cares for patients taking part in clinical trials. She has just finished her lunch break and has returned to care for her patient in the critical care department. Her patient, Mr Harif, is being treated with an experimental medication to treat COVID pneumonitis as part of a trial. This requires careful monitoring to ensure that the medication does not cause harmful side effects or fail to produce positive clinical outcomes. During the rest of the afternoon Susan is extremely busy and doesn't get a chance to complete her nursing documentation. By the time she finds time to complete her documentation, she feels there is no time to write it all from scratch, so uses the digital

(Continued)

(Continued)

record system to 'copy and paste' sections of documentation from the previous day into the record for her shift. Without realising, Susan inadvertently copies across documentation indicating that Mr Harif was experiencing side effects from the experimental medication which he was actually no longer experiencing. She also copied across documentation indicating that Mr Harif had other symptoms which had now improved.

Activity 7.2   Reflection

What could the impacts on Mr Harif be in this case study? Reflect on what this scenario tells us about the nature of digital clinical data.

An outline answer is provided at the end of this chapter.

Chapter summary

This chapter has explored digital innovation in nursing practice, including key innovations in digital nursing practice which have benefitted patients. In addition, the potential unintended consequences of digital innovation have been explored alongside the importance of effective management of digital data.

Innovations in digital health technologies have enormous potential to improve patient care and increase opportunities to conduct research on increasingly large cohorts of participants. These innovations may also save time and improve access to reliable health information for both professionals and patients.

Maximising the potential of digital innovations requires nurses to adopt a critical approach to the selection, adoption and implementation of technologies and use of digital sources of information. It is essential that nurses remain cognisant of the complex ethical challenges associated with digital technologies, information and clinical data.

Activities: brief outline answers

Activity 7.1   Reflection (page 106)

You need to establish the answers to two clinical questions. First, what preventative interventions are required? Second, which dressings are most appropriate for the grade IV pressure ulcer? You could obtain information from the following sources: local policies accessible via the local 'intranet'. The intranet is a computer network for sharing information and other computing services within an organisation. Alternatively, you could obtain evidence-based clinical guidance from a reputable online source such as the National Institute for Health and Care Excellence

(NICE) which publishes evidence-based guidelines. After reviewing the local policy and the NICE guidance, you identify the preventative interventions needed in Miss Jennings's case. In addition, you read that a referral to a tissue viability nurse (TVN) for specialist input is appropriate. Following the provision of guidance from the TVN, any recommended dressing products could be looked up in the British National Formulary online site. This would provide information related to any contraindications to using the dressings which you may need to be aware of.

Activity 7.2   Reflection (page 110)

The nature of digital clinical records is unique in that large sections of data can be copied instantaneously and uncritically. This is unlike handwritten records which would need to be read prior to any copying that might mitigate the risks of this scenario occurring. Evidence indicates that copy and pasting digital health records may lead to note bloat, internal inconsistencies, error propagation and documentation in the wrong patient records (Tsou et al., 2017). Misrecording nursing documentation by inappropriately copying old clinical documentation using a digital system may cause Mr Harif to be subject to further medical treatment which he does not require, or have experimental medication withdrawn which could have been helping him. This directly contravenes the core ethical principles of beneficence and non-maleficence. In addition, the data analysed as part of the clinical trial will be undermined which could have negative impacts. Over time, if data was continuously mishandled in this way, the negative impacts on both individual patients and on our understanding of the efficacy of care could be significant, and ultimately to the detriment of patients.

Chapter 8 Your ongoing digital development

Emma Gillaspy

HEE Digital Capabilities Framework

This book is intended to be used by student and registered nurses, and those supporting them to improve digital competencies. It is shaped using the Health and Care Digital Capability Framework, which we first saw in Chapter 1 (Figure 8.1).

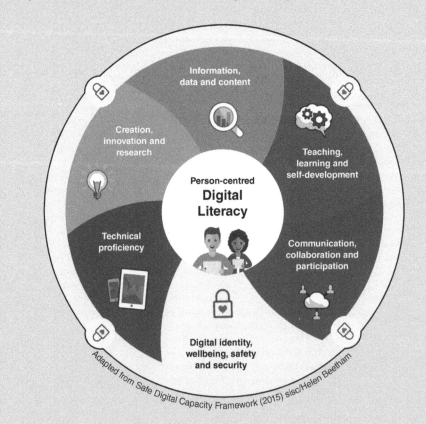

Figure 8.1 Health and Care Digital Capability Framework (Health Education England, 2018)

The framework includes six domains and progression through four different levels of digital capability. Each chapter is mapped against specific domains, providing the learner with a level 2 in digital capability. This chapter summarises the key learning points, focusing on the acquired knowledge and contribution to your professional identity as nurses.

Chapter aims

After reading this chapter, you will be able to:

- reflect on your digital capability development so far;
- consider how your digital skills and knowledge of digital health can improve your practice as a professional nurse;
- develop a plan to further your digital capabilities.

Introduction

This chapter summarises the key learning points across all the chapters in this book. You will first identify what you have learnt from your explorations in each chapter and how this will contribute to your professional identity as nurses. Using the common solutions-focused coaching model OSKAR, you will then identify personal objectives for the development of your digital capabilities in relation to your future nursing practice. You can repeat this activity at key times during your career – for example, during your revalidation or when preparing for a promotion. The reflective activities presented here focus on digital capability. However, you could equally apply this flexible process to examine other areas of your professional practice and personal development. You could also use this approach to empower your patients to take control of improving their health, or to support the development of your colleagues and teams.

Coaching for self-development

Coaching has been shown to reduce stress and improve well-being and resilience (Grover and Furnham, 2016) and is being widely advocated across health and social care settings. For example, we recommend the following resources:

- The NHS Leadership Academy highlights the benefits of a coaching approach to leadership, and lists regional coaching and mentoring offers on their resources website: www.leadershipacademy.nhs.uk/resources/coaching-register
- NHS England offer free coaching for staff in certain roles too: www.england.nhs.uk/supporting-our-nhs-people/support-now

- Have a read through some of the case studies to see how their coaching services have benefitted staff in primary care settings: www.employment-studies.co.uk/research-collections/looking-after-you-%E2%80%93-primary-care-coaching-case-studies
- Health coaching is also a supported self-management approach advocated by NHS England to help people achieve their health and well-being goals: www.england.nhs.uk/personalisedcare/supported-self-management/health-and-wellbeing-coaches

If you are interested in learning more about how coaching can help you develop, search for coaching services offered by your local employer or even learn to be a coach yourself through one of the many courses supported by health and social care organisations.

Why use the OSKAR coaching framework?

OSKAR is a popular solutions-focused coaching framework. It helps you to explore possibilities and solutions rather than focusing on the problem or what needs to be fixed. OSKAR was developed by coaches McKergow and Jackson (2006) and is based on an appreciative enquiry approach (Cooperrider et al., 2004) in which you find what works for you and do more of that. You may see similarities in this approach and clinical practices such as motivational interviewing, Cognitive Behavioural Therapy and Solution-focused Brief Therapy, so learning to look at your own strengths in this way will help you to support your patients too.

The OSKAR framework consists of five steps that can be repeated through a cyclical reflective process outlined in Figure 8.2:

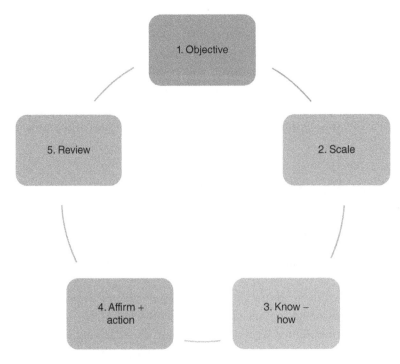

Figure 8.2   Five steps in the OSKAR coaching framework

When considering your ongoing digital development in this chapter, you will:

1. Identify an *objective* or desired outcome for your digital capability.

2. Quantify your current practice in each area of digital capability using a *scale* of 1–10.

3. Consider what *know-how* (knowledge, skills, attributes or resources) you will need to successfully reach your desired outcome.

4. Reflect on your strengths (*affirm*) and how these can be leveraged to take positive *action* towards your goal.

5. Identify measures to review your ongoing progress and consider how this will impact on your professional development as a digitally enabled nurse.

Activity 8.1   Identifying your desired outcome

Reflecting on your current practice and the ideas you have explored throughout this book, can you identify a new overall goal you would like to achieve for your digital capability as a nurse? For example, this could be building your confidence further, practising your digital skills or using digital health approaches with your patients. What kind of digitally enabled nurse do you want to become and why is this important to you? Write this goal down in the space below.

My overall goal for digital development is:

....

....

....

Tip: to help you in completing this activity, you may wish to return to the links in Activity 1.2 and repeat your chosen self-assessment. Remember you can return to this at any time in your career.

As this activity is based on your own reflection, no answer is given at the end of this chapter.

Activity 8.2   Quantifying your current practice

Looking back through each chapter of this book and thinking about your overarching goal for development from Activity 8.1, if you were to score each of these areas a perfect 10 out of 10, can you describe what that would look like for you? Write this down, either as a list or on a wheel. We have illustrated an example for your digital toolkit below. Remember everyone's perfect 10 is different, so think about what this means for you.

Now give yourself a score for each area out of 10 where the centre of the wheel is zero (not at all effective) and the outer edge is 10 (highly effective). Remember, this is in the context of the overall desired outcome you wrote for Activity 8.1. Here's an example of what your scores might look like.

(Continued)

(Continued)

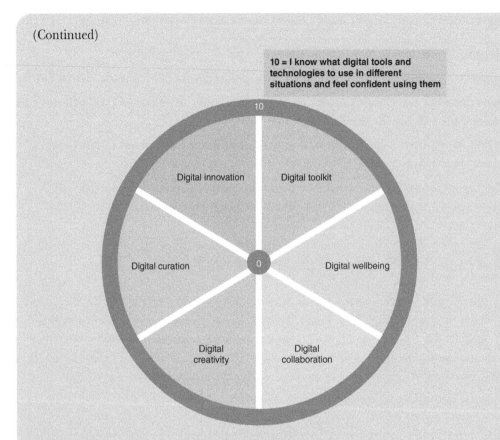

Figure 8.3 Goals for development template

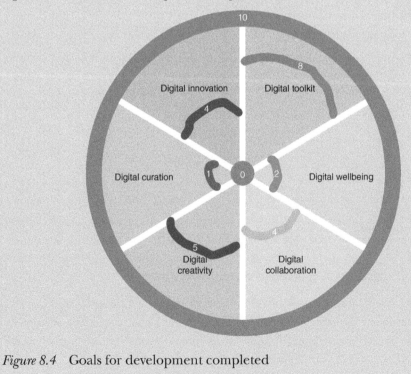

Figure 8.4 Goals for development completed

Finally, pick one area that is the most important for you to change soon.

My top priority for digital development is:

....

As this activity is based on your own reflection, no outline answer is given at the end of this chapter.

Activity 8.3   Your know-how

Taking the top priority for you, write down what the next score up would look like. For example, if I chose digital well-being, I would describe what a score of 3 would look like. You wouldn't expect to ride a bike the first time you get on one, so try not to think about how to get to your perfect 10 in an area, just think about the next score up – or even half score if that feels too much.

For my priority area of .... , the next score up of

.... would look like

....

....

What skills, knowledge, attributes do you need to reach the next score up?

Skills ....

Knowledge ....

Attributes ....

What else? ....

As this activity is based on your own reflection, no outline answer is given at the end of this chapter.

Activity 8.4   Affirm and action

Affirm (what is already going well): consider some of the following reflective questions in relation to developing this priority area:

*   What strengths do you already have that you can draw upon to develop this area?
*   What are you already doing to achieve the score you have given yourself? Could you do more of this?

(Continued)

(Continued)

Action (what are you going to do):

- What will you do as a first step towards the next score? Does this feel doable? If not, can you break the step into smaller chunks? The key here is for your first step to feel achievable, then, when you complete it, it will give you the motivation to continue your success.
- When are you going to do it? Try to include an exact time and date and ideally tell someone about it. This will make your action more likely to happen.
- What might get in the way of you achieving this next step? What could you do to mitigate this potential barrier?
- Do you need anything (e.g., support, time, resources) to make it happen? How are you going to make sure you seek what you need?

As this activity is based on your own reflection, no outline answer is given at the end of this chapter.

Activity 8.5   Review

Now put a date in your diary when you are going to come back and review your progress – this could be as a reminder on your phone, on your digital or even physical calendar.

- How will you evaluate if you have been successful? Add as much detail as you can now so that when you see your reminder, you remember the progress you expected to see.
- Ask yourself 'what next?' You can go back to your scored wheel in activity 8.2 and focus on developing your next priority. Or you may choose to further your development in the same area.

As this activity is based on your own reflection, no outline answer is given at the end of this chapter.

Activity 8.6   Reflection on the process

Have a think about the self-coaching process of development planning that you have been through in this chapter. What other areas of your professional or personal practice could benefit from a similar process? How could you use this technique with patients to help them manage their health more independently?

Challenge: can you share this process with one other person who you think this might be beneficial for?

As this activity is based on your own reflection, no outline answer is given at the end of this chapter.

Chapter summary

This chapter has encouraged you to reflect on all the elements of the previous chapters and outline a personal plan for further development. A commonly used coaching model was used to structure the chapter to provide a way for you to consider your goals and priorities in a meaningful, timely and personalised way. It is hoped that by completing this self-coaching process, you are learning a vital skill which you can apply, not just to develop your digital capability, but across your nursing studies and future practice. We hope you have enjoyed reading this book and have gained an understanding of how digital capability is core to the skills of a professional nurse.

References

Alanazi, A., Alomar, M., Aldosari, H., Shahrani, A. and Aldosari, B. (2018) The effect of electronic medication administration records on the culture of patient safety: a literature review. *Studies in Health Technology and Informatics*, 251: 223–6.

AMRC (2020) Navigating the digital health ethics landscape: a framework for understanding ethical principles for digital health. Available at: www.amrc.org.uk/navigating-the-digital-health-ethics-landscape-a-framework-for-understanding-ethical-principles-for-digital-health (accessed 12 September 2022).

Andrews, H., Tierney, S. and Seers, K. (2020) Needing permission: the experience of self-care and self-compassion in nursing: a constructivist grounded theory study. *International Journal of Nursing Studies*, 101: 103436. Available at: https://doi.org/10.1186/s12889-021-12169-7 (accessed 24 November 2022).

Association of Internet Researchers (AIOR) with Franzke, Aline Shakti, Bechmann, Anja, Zimmer, Michael, Ess, Charles (2020) *Internet Research: Ethical Guidelines 3.0.* Available at https://aoir.org/reports/ethics3.pdf

Awori, J. and Lee, J.M. (2017) A maker movement for health: a new paradigm for health innovation. *JAMA Pediatrics*, 171 (2): 107–8. Available at: https://doi.org/10.1001/jamapediatrics.2016.3747

Bailey, S. and Burhouse, A. (2019) From superhero to super-connector, changing the leadership culture in the NHS. *Future Healthcare Journal*, 6 (2): 106–9. Available at: https://doi.org/10.7861/futurehosp.6-2-106

Beckingham, S. (2019) Developing a professional online presence and effective network, in C. Rowell (ed.) *Social Media in Higher Education: Case Studies, Reflections and Analysis.* Cambridge: Open Book Publishers (pp. 21–34).

Brawanski, A. (2012) On the myth of the Edwin Smith papyrus: is it magic or science? *Acta Neurochirurgica*, 154 (12): 2285–91. Available at: https://doi.org/10.1007/s00701-012-1523-x

Brice, S. and Almond, H. (2020) Health professional digital capabilities frameworks: a scoping review. *Journal of Multidisciplinary Healthcare*, 13: 1375–90. Available at: https://doi.org/10.2147/jmdh.s269412

British Medical Association (2018) Access to health records: updated to reflect the General Data Protection Regulation and Data Protection Act 2018: Guidance for health professionals in the United Kingdom. Available at: www.bma.org.uk/media/2821/bma-access-to-health-records-june-20.pdf (accessed 12 October 2022).

Brits, H., Botha, A., Niksch, L., Terblanché, R., Venter, K. and Joubert, G. (2017) Illegible handwriting and other prescription errors on prescriptions at National District Hospital, Bloemfontein. *Professional Nursing Today*, 21 (2): 53–6.

Brod, C. (1984) *Technostress: The Human Cost of the Computer Revolution.* Reading, MA: Longman.

Brooks, B.A. (2014) An emerging role: the nurse content curator. *Nursing Forum.* 50 (1): 51–4.

Brown, J., Pope, N., Bosco, A. M., Mason, J., and Morgan, A. (2020) Issues affecting nurses' capability to use digital technology at work: an integrative review. *Journal of Clinical Nursing*, 29 (15–16): 2801–19.

Buck, S. (2013) If you use the Web, you are a "curator." Available at: http://mashable.com/2013/05/09/curator (accessed 18 August 2022).

Carers Trust (2015) About caring. Available at: https://carers.org/about-caring/about-caring (accessed 10 August 2022).

Carers UK (2021) State of caring 2021: a snapshot of unpaid care in the UK. Available at: www.carersuk.org/images/Research/CUK_State_of_Caring_2021_report_web.pdf?_ga=2.44762348.998735536.1638353300-1463435790.1638353300 (accessed 10 August 2022).

Carretero, S., Vuorikari, R., and Punie, Y. (2017) *DigComp 2.1.* The digital competence framework for citizens with eight proficiency levels and examples of use. Available at: https://op.europa.eu/en/publication-detail/-/publication/3c5e7879-308f-11e7-9412-01aa75ed71a1/language-en (accessed 10 August 2022).

Cassidy, J.T., Fitzgerald, E., Cassidy, E.S., Cleary, M., Byrne, D.P., Devitt, B.M., Baker, J.F. (2018) YouTube provides poor information regarding anterior cruciate ligament injury and reconstruction. *Knee Surgery, Sports Traumatology, Arthroscopy*, 26: 840–5. Available at: https://doi.org/10.1007/s00167-017-4514-x (accessed 24 November 2022).

Claro, M., Preiss, D., San Martín, E., Jara, I., Hinostroza, J. Valenzüela, S. et al. (2012) Assessment of 21st century ICT skills in Chile: test design and results from high school level students. *Computers & Education*, 59 (3): 1042–53. Available at: https://doi.org/10.1016/j.compedu.2012.04.004 (accessed 24 November 2022).

Coalition for Personalised Care (2022) Co-production. Available at: https://www.coalitionforpersonalisedcare.org.uk/co-production (accessed 17 January 2023).

Cole, D., Rengasamy, E., Batchelor, S. et al. (2017) Using social media to support small group learning. *BMC Medical Education*, 17: 201. Available at: https://doi.org/10.1186/s12909-017-1060-7 (accessed 24 November 2022).

Conaty-Buck, S. (2017) Cybersecurity and healthcare records, *American Nurse Today*, 12 (9): 62–4.

Cooperrider, D.L., Whitney, D. Stavros, J.M. (eds) (2004) *Appreciative Inquiry Handbook: The first in a series of AI workbooks for leaders of change.* Oakland, CA: Berrett-Koehler.

Crompton, H. and Burke, D. (2018) The use of mobile learning in higher education: a systematic review, *Computers and Education*, 123: 53–64.

Dale, S. (2014) Content curation: the future of relevance. *Business Information Review*, 31 (4): 199–205.

Data Protection Act (2018) Available at: www.legislation.gov.uk/ukpga/2018/12/contents/enacted (accessed 14 September 2022).

Davies, J., Pucher, P.H., Ibrahim, H. and Stubbs, B. (2017) Impact of the introduction of electronic prescribing on staff perceptions of patient safety and organizational culture. *Journal of Surgical Research*, 212: 222–8. Available at: https://doi.org/10.1016/j.jss.2017.02.001 (accessed 24 November 2024).

Day-Calder, M. (2019) When friendly is too friendly, and knowing where to draw the line. *Nursing Standard*, 36 (12): 27–8. Available at: https://doi.org/10.7748/ns.36.12.27.s15 (accessed 24 November 2022).

Department for Education (2018) *Essential Digital Skills Framework*. Available at: https://assets.publishing.service.gov.uk/government/uploads/system/uploads/attachment_data/file/738922/Essential_digital_skills_framework.pdf (accessed 24 November 2022).

Department for Education and Skills (2003) *21st Century Skills: Realising our Potential*. Norwich: Stationery Office.

Department of Health (1991) *Patient's Charter*. London: Department of Health.

Department of Health (2022) Data saves lives: reshaping health and social care with data. Policy paper. Available at: www.gov.uk/government/publications/data-saves-lives-reshaping-health-and-social-care-with-data (accessed 24 November 2024).

Department of Health and Social Care (2021) A guide to good practice for digital and data-driven health technologies. Available at: https://www.gov.uk/government/publications/code-of-conduct-for-data-driven-health-and-care-technology/initial-code-of-conduct-for-data-driven-health-and-care-technology (accessed 15 July 2022)

Department of Health and Social Care (2021) Putting data, digital and tech at the heart of transforming the NHS. London: Department of Health and Social Care. Available at: www.gov.uk/government/publications/putting-data-digital-and-tech-at-the-heart-of-transforming-the-nhs/putting-data-digital-and-tech-at-the-heart-of-transforming-the-nhs#concluding-remarks (accessed 24 November 2022).

Dhar, V.K., Kim, Y., Graff, J.T. et al. (2018) Benefit of social media on patient engagement and satisfaction: results of a 9-month, qualitative pilot study using Facebook. *Surgery*, 163 (3): 565–70. Available at: https://doi.org/10.1016/j.surg.2017.09.056 (accessed 24 November 2022).

DigitalEurope (2021) A digital health decade: from ambition to action. Brussels. Available at: www.digitaleurope.org/wp/wp-content/uploads/2021/11/DIGITALEUROPE_A-digital-health-decade_From-ambition-to-action.pdf (accessed 24 November 2022).

Digital Health Laws and Regulations UK (2022) Available at: https://iclg.com/practice-areas/digital-health-laws-and-regulations/united-kingdom (accessed 24 November 2022).

EHTEL (2012) Ethical principles for eHealth. A briefing paper. Available at: https://archived.ehtel.eu/publications/position-andbriefing-papers/ETHICAL-briefing-principles-for-ehealth/view (accessed 12 August 2022).

Elliott, M. and Liu, Y. (2013) The nine rights of medication administration: an overview. *British Journal of Nursing*, 19 (5): 300–5. Available at: https://doi.org/10.12968/bjon.2010.19.5.47064 (accessed 24 November 2022).

European Commission (2018) Consultation: transformation health and care in the digital single market. European Union. Available at: https://ec.europa.eu/health/sites/default/files/ehealth/docs/2018_consultation_dsm_en.pdf (accessed 12 July 2022).

European Schoolnet (2016) The e-Skills Manifesto. Belgium. Available at: http://www.eun.org/documents/411753/817341/eSkills_Manifesto_2016.pdf/6a1ac5e4-2409-4f33-ace1-81fc689956ec (accessed 24 November 2022).

Featherall, J., Lapin B., Chaitoff A., Havele S.A., Thompson N. and Katzan I. (2018) Characterization of patient interest in provider-based consumer health information technology: survey study. *Journal of Medical Internet Research*. 20: e128. Available at: https://doi.org/10.2196/jmir.7766 (accessed 24 November 2022).

Fielding, J.A. (2019) Rethinking CRAAP: getting students thinking like fact-checkers in evaluating web sources, *College & Research Libraries News*, 80 (11): 620–2. Available at: https://doi.org/10.5860/crln.80.11.620 (accessed 24 November 2022).

Flintoff, K., Mellow, P. and Clark, K.P. (2014) *Digital Curation: Opportunities for Learning, Teaching, Research and Professional Development. Conference: 23rd Annual Teaching and Learning Forum.* Perth, University of Western Australia

Flynn, G.A.H., Polivka, B. and Behr, J.H. (2018) Smartphone use by nurses in acute care settings, CIN: *Computers, Informatics, Nursing*, 36 (3): 120–6. Available at: https://doi.org/10.1097/cin.0000000000000400 (accessed 24 November 2022).

Francis, R. (2013) *Report of the Mid Staffordshire NHS Foundation Trust Public Inquiry* (1st edn [ebook]). London: Robert Francis, p. 1168. Available at: https://assets.publishing.service.gov.uk/government/uploads/system/uploads/attachment_data/file/279118/0898_ii.pdf (accessed 24 November 2022).

Gaba, D. (2004) The future vision of simulation in health care. *Quality and Safety in Healthcare*. 13 (1): 2–10.

Gabarron, E., Oyeyemi, S.O. and Wynn, R. (2021) COVID-19-related misinformation on social media: a systematic review. *Bulletin of the World Health Organization*, 99 (6): 455–63A. Available at: https://doi.org/10.2471/BLT.20.276782 (accessed 24 November 2022).

Gabbard G.O. (2019) Digital professionalism. *Academic Psychiatry*. 43 (3): 259–63.

Ganasegeran, K. and Abdulrahman, S.A. (2019) Adopting m-health in clinical practice: a boon or a bane? *Telemedicine Technologies*, pp. 31–41. Available at: https://doi.org/10.1016/B978-0-12-816948-3.00003-9 (accessed 24 November 2022).

Garner, J., Gillaspy, E., Smith, M., Blackburn, C., Craddock, A., Drew, T., Holmes, S., Jones, R. and anonymous service user (2022) Co-producing nurse education with academics, students, service users and carers: lessons from the pandemic. *British Journal of Nursing*, 31 (16): 854–60. Available at: https://doi.org/10.12968/bjon.2022.31.16.854 (accessed 24 November 2022).

Gates, P.J., Hardie, R.-A., Raban, M.Z., Li, L. and Westbrook, J.I. (2020) How effective are electronic medication systems in reducing medication error rates and associated harm among hospital inpatients? A systematic review and meta-analysis. *Journal of the American Medical Informatics Association*, 28 (1): 167–76. Available at: https://doi.org/10.1093/jamia/ocaa230 (accessed 24 November 2022).

Gillaspy, E. and Vasilica, C. (2021) Developing the digital self-determined learner through heutagogical design. *Higher Education Pedagogies*, 6 (1): 135–55. Available at: https://doi.org/10.1080/23752696.2021.1916981 (accessed 24 November 2022).

Google (2020) Digital wellbeing. Available at: https://wellbeing.google/ (accessed 24 November 2022).

Goundrey-Smith, S.J. (2019) Technologies that transform: digital solutions for optimising medicines use in the NHS. *BMJ Health & Care Informatics*, 26 (1). Available at: https://doi.org/10.1136/bmjhci-2019-100016 (accessed 24 November 2022).

Gray, K. and Sockolow, P. (2016) Conceptual models in health informatics research: a literature review and suggestions for development. *JMIR Medical Informatics*, 4 (1).

Greenhalgh, T., Wherton, J., Shaw, S. and Morrison, C. (2020) Video consultations for Covid-19. *British Medical Journal*. Available at: https://doi.org/10.1136/bmj.m998 (accessed 24 November 2022).

Grover, S. and Furnham, A. (2016) Coaching as a developmental intervention in organisations: a systematic review of its effectiveness and the mechanisms underlying it. *PLoS ONE*, 11 (7): e0159137.

Guk, K., Han, G., Lim, J., Jeong, K., Kang, T., Lim, E-K. and Jung, J. (2019) Evolution of wearable devices with real-time disease monitoring for personalized healthcare. *Nanomaterials*, 9 (6): 813. Available at: https://doi.org/10.3390/nano90608

Guallar, J. (2020) Personal content curator system: steps, tools and examples. Proceedings of the On Topic, Zaragoza, Spain.

Guallar, J. (2021) *Los Content Curators: Toolkit Content Curator*. Available at: www.loscontentcurators.com/toolkitcontent-curator-edicion-2022/ (accessed 24 Novmber 2022).

Guo, C., Ashrafian, H., Ghafur, S., Fontana, G., Gardner, C., and Prime, M. (2020) Challenges for the evaluation of digital health solutions – a call for innovative evidence generation approaches. *npj Digital Medicine*, 3: 110. Available at: https://doi.org/10.1038/s41746-020-00314-2 (accessed 24 November 2022).

Guraya, S.S., Guraya, Y.S. and Yusoff, B.S.M. (2021) Preserving professional identities, behaviors, and values in digital professionalism using social networking sites; a systematic review. *BMC Medical Education*, 21: 381. Available at: https://doi.org/10.1186/s12909-021-02802-9

Haslam, M.B. (2020) How virtual communities of practice via social media might enhance nurse education. *The Journal of Social Media for Learning*, 1 (1).

Hazara, A., Durrans, K. and Bhandari, S. (2019) The role of patient portals in enhancing self-care in patients with renal conditions. *Clinical Kidney Journal*, 13 (1): 1–7. Available at: https://doi.org/10.1093/ckj/sfz154

Health Education England (HEE) (2018) *A Health and Care Digital Capabilities Framework*. London: HEE.

Huhman, H. (2011) Skillset vs. mindset: which will get you the job? *[blog]*. Available at: https://money.usnews.com/money/blogs/outside-voices-careers/2011/08/26/skillset-vs-mindset-which-will-get-you-the-job (accessed 24 November 2022).

Hwang, J.-I. and Park, H.-A. (2011) Factors associated with nurses' informatics competency. *CIN: Computers, Informatics, Nursing*, 29 (4): 256–62. Available at: https://doi.org/10.1097/NCN.0b013e3181fc3d24 (accessed 24 November 2022).

Iyawa, G.E., Herselman, M. and Botha, A. (2016) Digital health innovation ecosystems: from systematic literature review to conceptual framework. *Procedia Computer Science*, 100: 244–52. Available at: https://doi.org/10.1016/j.procs.2016.09.149 (accessed 24 November 2022).

Jacob, P.D. (2020) Management of patient healthcare information: healthcare-related information flow, access, and availability. *Fundamentals of Telemedicine and Telehealth*, pp. 35–57. Available at: https://doi.org/10.1016/B978-0-12-814309-4.00003-3 (accessed 24 November 2022).

Jain, N., Abboudi, H., Kalic, A., Gill, F., Al-Hasani, H. (2019) YouTube as a source of patient information for transrectal ultrasound-guided biopsy of the prostate. *Clinical Radiology*, 74 (79): e11–79. e14.

Jandoo, T. (2020) WHO guidance for digital health: what it means for researchers. *Digital Health*, 6. Available at: https://doi.org/10.1177/2055207619898984 (accessed 24 November 2022).

Jenkins, H., Purushotma, R., Weigel, M., Clinton, K. and Robinson, A.J. (2009) *Confronting the Challenges of Participatory Culture: Media Education for the 21st Century: A Report for the MacArthur Foundatio*n. Boston, MA: MIT Press.

Jin, K., Khonsari, S., Gallagher, R., Gallagher, P., Clark, A.M., Freedman, B., Briffa, T., Bauman, A., Redfern, J. and Neubeck, L. (2019) Telehealth interventions for the secondary prevention of coronary heart disease: a systematic review and meta-analysis. *European Journal of Cardiovascular Nursing*, 18 (4): 260–71. Available at: https://doi.org/10.1177/1474515119826510 (accessed 24 November 2022).

JISC (2015) Individual digital capabilities. Available at: https://digitalcapability.jisc.ac.uk/what-is-digital-capability/individual-digital-capabilities/ (accessed 24 November 2022).

JISC (2019) Digital wellbeing. Available at: https://digitalcapability.jisc.ac.uk/what-is-digital-capability/digital-wellbeing/ (accessed 24 November 2022).

Kata, A. (2012) Anti-vaccine activists, Web 2.0, and the postmodern paradigm – an overview of tactics and tropes used online by the anti-vaccination movement. *Vaccine*, 30 (25): 3778–89.

Keykaleh, S.M., Sarfarpour, H., Yousefian, S., Faghisolouk, F., Mohammadi, E. and Ghomian, Z. (2018) The relationship between nurse's job stress and patient safety. *Macedonian Journal of Medical Sciences*, 6 (11): 228–32. Available at: https://dx.doi.org/10.3889%2Foamjms2018.351.

Khodaveisi, T., Sadoughi, F. and Novin, K. (2020) Required data elements and requirements of a eleoncology system to provide treatment plans for patients with breast cancer. *International Journal of Cancer Management*, 13: 1–14. Available at: https://doi.org/10.5812/ijcm.100522 (accessed 24 November 2022).

Kim, J.U. and Park, H. (2019) Effects of smartphone-based mobile learning in nursing education: a systematic review and meta-analysis. *Asian Nursing Research*, 13 (1): 20–9.

Kim, J.U., Shin, H., Lee, J., Kang, S. and Bartlett, R. (2017) A smartphone application to educate undergraduate nursing students about providing care for infant airway obstruction. *Nurse Education Today*, 48: 145–52.

Kirschner, P.A. and de Bruyckere, P. (2017) The myths of the digital native and the multitasker. *Teaching and Teacher Education*, 67: 135–42. Available at: https://doi.org/10.1016/j.tate.2017.06.001 (accessed 24 November 2022).

Kispeter, E. (2018) Digital skills and inclusion research working group evidence brief. *Warwick Institute for Employment Research, University of Warwick*. Available at: https://assets.publishing.service.gov.uk/government/uploads/system/uploads/attachment_data/file/807831/What_digital_skills_do_adults_need_to_succeed_in_the_workplace_now_and_in_the_next_10_years_.pdf (accessed 24 November 2022).

Kleib, M. and Nagle, L. (2018) Factors associated with Canadian nurses' informatics competency. *CIN: Computers, Informatics, Nursing*, 36 (8): 406–15. Available at: https://doi.org/10.3928/00220124-20100503-08 (accessed 20 November 2022).

Kobayashi, R. and Ishizaki, M. (2019) Examining the interaction between medical information seeking online and understanding: exploratory study. *JMIR Cancer.* Available at: https://doi.org/10.2196/13240 (accessed 24 November 2022).

Kremer, H., Villamor, I. and Aguinis, H. (2019) Innovation leadership: best-practice recommendations for promoting employee creativity, voice, and knowledge sharing. *Business Horizons,* 62: 65–74.

Kumar, P., Sammut, S.M., Madan, J.J., Bucher, S. and Brice Kumar, M. (2021) Digital ≠ paperless: novel interfaces needed to address global health challenges. *BMJ Global Health* 2021. Available at: https://doi.org/10.1136/bmjgh-2021-005780 (accessed 24 November 2022).

Lachman, V.D. (2013) Social media: managing the ethical issues. *MedSurg Nursing,* 22 (5): 326–9.

Lave, J. and Wenger, E. (1991) *Situated Learning: Legitimate Peripheral Participation.* New York: Cambridge University Press.

Lederman, R., Kurnia, S., Peng, F. and Dreyfus, S. (2015) Tick a box, any box: a case study on the unintended consequences of system misuse in a hospital emergency department. *Journal of Information Technology Teaching Cases,* 5 (2): 74–83. Available at: https://doi.org/10.1057/jittc.2015.13 (accessed 24 November 2022).

Mackey, T.P. and Jacobson, T.E. (2011) Reframing information literacy as a metaliteracy. *College & Research Libraries,* 72 (1) 62–78. Available at: https://doi.org/10.5860/crl-76r1 (accessed 24 November 2022).

Macmillan Dictionary (2014) content curation. Available at: www.macmillandictionary.com/us/opendictionary/entries/content-curation.htm (accessed 12 August 2022).

Madrigal, L. and Escoffery, C. (2019) Electronic health behaviors among US adults with chronic disease: cross-sectional survey. *Journal of Medical Internet Research,* 21 (3). Available at: https://doi.org/10.2196/11240 (accessed 24 November 2022).

Marar, S.D., Al-Madaney M.M. and Almousawi, F.H. (2019) Health information on social media. *Saudi Medical Journal,* 40: 1294–8. Available at: https://doi.org/10.15537/smj.2019.12.24682 (accessed 24 November 2022).

Marcu A., Muller C., Ream E. and Whitaker K.L. (2019) Online information-seeking about potential breast cancer symptoms: capturing online behavior with an internet browsing tracking tool. *Journal of Medical Internet Research.* 21: e12400. Available at: https://doi.org/10.2196/12400 (accessed 24 November 2022).

Mariano, B. (2020) Towards a global strategy on digital health. *Bulletin of the World Health Organization,* 98 (4): 231–31A. Available at: https://doi.org/10.2471/blt.20.253955 (accessed 24 November 2022).

McKeown, M., Malihi-Shoja, L. and Downe, S., supporting the Comensus writing collective (2010) *Service User and Carer Involvement in Education for Health and Social Care.* Wiley-Blackwell.

McKergow and Jackson (2006) *The Solutions Focus: Making Coaching and Change Simple* (2nd edn). London: Nicholas Brealey.

Mehrotra, A., Paone, S., Martich, G.D., Albert, S.M. and Shevchik, G.J. (2013) A comparison of care at e-visits and physician office visits for sinusitis and urinary tract infection. *JAMA Internal Medicine,* 173 (1): 72–4. Available at: https://doi.org/10.1001/2013.jamainternmed.305 (accessed 24 November 2022).

Menon, A.K., Jiang, X., Kim, J., Vaidya, J. and Ohno-Machado, L. (2014) Detecting inappropriate access to electronic health records using collaborative filtering. *Machine Learning*, 95 (1): 87–101.

Merolli, M., Gray, K. and Martin-Sanchez, F. (2013) Health outcomes and related effects of using social media in chronic disease management: a literature review and analysis of affordances. *Journal Biomedical Information*, 46 (6): 957–69.

Merriam-Webster Online Dictionary (2014) *curator*. Available at: www.merriam-webster.com/ (accessed 17 August 2022).

Meskó, B., Drobni, Z., Bényei, É., Gergely, B. and Győrffy, Z. (2017) Digital health is a cultural transformation of traditional healthcare. *mHealth*, 3: 38–38. Available at: https://doi.org/10.21037/mhealth.2017.08.07 (accessed 24 November 2022).

Minocha, S. and Petre, M. (2012) *Handbook of Social Media for Researchers and Supervisors.* London: Sage.

Monteiro, C., Avelar, M.F.A. and da Luz Goncalves Pedreira, M. (2017) Interruptions of nurses' activities and patient safety: an integrative literature review. *Revista Latino – Americana De Enfermagem*, 23 (1): 169–79. Available at: https://dx.doi.org/10.1590%2F0104-1169.0251.2539 (accessed 24 November 2022).

Mukoro, F. (2012) *Renal Patient View – A System Which Provides Patients Online Access to Their Test Results. Final Evaluation Report.* London: Department of Health.

National Commission for the Protection of Human Subjects of Biomedical and Behavioral Research (1979) *The Belmont Report: ethical principles and guidelines for the protection of human subjects of research.* Available at: www.hhs.gov/ohrp/regulations-and-policy/belmont-report/index.html (accessed 24 November 2022).

National Cyber Security Agency (2020) What is cybersecurity? Available at: www.ncsc.gov.uk/section/about-ncsc/what-is-cyber-security (accessed 24 November 2022).

National Health Service (NHS) The NHS Long Term Plan (2019) Available at: www.longtermplan.nhs.uk/wp-content/uploads/2019/08/nhs-long-term-plan-version-1.2.pdf (accessed 24 November 2022).

Navarro Martínez, O., Igual García, J. and Traver Salcedo, V. (2021) Estimating patient empowerment and nurses' use of digital strategies: eSurvey study. *International Journal of Environmental Research and Public Health*, 18 (18): 9844.

Nazeha, N., Pavagadhi, D., Kyaw, B., Car, J., Jimenez, G. and Tudor Car, L. (2020) A digitally competent health workforce: scoping review of educational frameworks. *Journal of Medical Internet Research*, 22 (11). Available at: https://doi.org/10.2196/22706 (accessed 24 November 2022).

Nebeker, C., Torus, J., and Bartlett Ellis, R.J. (2019) Building the case for actionable ethics in digital health research supported by artificial intelligence. *BMC Medicine* 17 (137). Available at: https://doi.org/10.1186/s12916-019-1377-7

NHS Digital (2022) Why digital inclusion matters to health and social care. Available at: https://digital.nhs.uk/about-nhs-digital/our-work/digital-inclusion/digital-inclusion-in-health-and-social-care#document-content

NHS Digital Academy (2021) Digital transformation. Available at: https://digital-transformation.hee.nhs.uk/digital-academy/ (accessed 24 November 2022).

NHS England (2021) Integration and innovation: working together to improve health and social care for all. White Paper. Available at: www.gov.uk/government/publications/working-together-to-improve-health-and-social-care-for-all/integration-and-innovation-working-together-to-improve-health-and-social-care-for-all-html-version (accessed 24 November 2022).

NHS Health Education England (2016) *Make Every Contact Count.* Available at: www.makingeverycontactcount.co.uk/ (accessed 24 November 2022).

NICE (2022) *Evidence Standards Framework for Digital Health Technologies.* Available at: www.nice.org.uk/corporate/ecd7 (accessed 24 November 2022).

Nursing and Midwifery Council (2018a) *The Code: Professional Standards of Practice and Behaviour for Nurses, Midwives and Nursing Associates.* Available at: www.nmc.org.uk/standards/code/ (accessed 24 November 2022).

Nursing and Midwifery Council (2018b) *Standards of Proficiency for Registered Nurses.* Available at: www.nmc.org.uk/standards/standards-for-nurses/standards-of-proficiency-for-registered-nurses/ (accessed 24 November 2022).

Nursing and Midwifery Council (2019) *Guidance on Using Social Media Responsibly.* Available at: www.nmc.org.uk/standards/guidance/social-media-guidance/ accessed 24 November 2022).

Nursing and Midwifery Council (2020) *NMC Guidance During the Covid-19 Emergency Period.* Available at: www.nmc.org.uk/globalassets/sitedocuments/ftp_information/nmc-guidance-during-the-covid-19-emergency-period.pdf (accessed 24 November 2022).

Nursing and Midwifery Council (2022) *Current Recovery Programme Standards.* Available at: www.nmc.org.uk/globalassets/sitedocuments/education-standards/current-recovery-programme-standards.pdf (accessed 24 November 2022).

O'Connor, S. and Andrews, T. (2018) Smartphones and mobile applications (apps) in clinical nursing education: a student perspective. *Nurse Education Today*, 69: 172–8. Available at: https://doi.org/10.1016/j.nedt.2018.07.013 (accessed 24 November 2022).

Office for National Statistics (2021) Exploring the UK's digital divide. Available at: www.ons.gov.uk/peoplepopulationandcommunity/householdcharacteristics/homeinternetandsocialmediausage/articles/exploringtheuksdigitaldivide/2019-03-04 (accessed 24 November 2022).

Oliver, J., Dutch, M., Rojek, A., Putland, M. and Knott, J. (2022) Remote COVID-19 patient monitoring system: a qualitative evaluation. *BMJ Open*, 12 (5): e054601. Available at: https://doi.org/10.1136/bmjopen-2021-054601 (accessed 24 November 2022).

O'Reilly, M. (2020) Social media and adolescent mental health: the good, the bad and the ugly. *Journal of Mental Health*, 29 (2): 200–6. Available at: https://doi.org/10.1080/09638237.2020.1714007

O'Reilly, M., Dogra, N., Hughes, J., Reilly, P., George, R. and Whiteman, N. (2019) Potential of social media in promoting mental health in adolescents. *Health Promotion International*, 34 (5): 981–91. Available at: https://doi.org/10.1093%2Fheapro%2Fday056 (accessed 24 November 2023).

Ostashewski, N., Andrew, B. and Romana, M. (2014) *Blended Learning and Digital Curation: A Course Activity Design Encouraging Student Engagement and Developing Critical Analysis Skills.* Proceedings of the EdMedia: World Conference on Educational Media and Technology, Tampere, Finlandia. Available at: https://www.editlib.org/p/147792/ (accessed 24 November 2022).

Oxford English Dictionary (2021) *Well-being*. Oxford: Oxford University Press.

Ramney, M., Patena, J., Nugent, N., Spirito, A.M., Boyer, E., Zatzick, D., Cunningham, R. (2016) PTSD, Cyberbullying and peer violence: prevalence and correlates among adolescent emergency department patients. *General Hospital Psychiatry*, 39. Available at: https://dx.doi.org/10.1016%2Fj.genhosppsych.2015.12.002 (accessed 24 November 2020).

Rawassizadeh, R., Price, B.A. and Petre, M. (2015) Wearables: has the age of smartwatches finally arrived? *Communications of the ACM*, 58: 45–7. Available at: https://doi.org/10.1145/2629633 (accessed 24 November 2022).

Reig, D. (2010) *Content Curator, Intermediario del Conocimiento: Nueva Profesión para la Web 3.0. El Caparazó*n. Available at: www.dreig.eu/caparazon/2010/01/09/content-curator-web-3/ (accessed 24 November 2022).

Resnik, D.B. (2015) What is ethics in research and why is it important? Available at: www.niehs.nih.gov/research/resources/bioethics/whatis/index.cfm (accessed 24 November 2022).

Rich, E., Lewis, S., Lupton, D., Miah, A. and Piwek, L. (2020) *Digital Health Generation?: Young People's Use of 'Healthy Lifestyle' Technologies*. Bath: University of Bath.

Robinson, K. and Webber, M. (2013) Models and effectiveness of service user and carer involvement in social work education: A literature review. *British Journal of Social Work*, 43 (5): 925–44.

Royal College of Nursing (2018) *Every Nurse an E-nurse*. London: Royal College of Nursing. Available at: www.rcn.org.uk/professional-development/publications/pdf-007013 (accessed 24 November 2022).

Royal Pharmaceutical Society (2019) *Professional guidance on the safe and secure handling of medicines* Available at: www.rpharms.com/recognition/setting-professional-standards/safe-and-secure-handling-of-medicines/professional-guidance-on-the-safe-and-secure-handling-of-medicines (accessed 24 November 2022).

Saab, M.M., Landers, M., Egan, S., Murphy, D. and Hegarty, J. (2021) Nurses and nursing students' attitudes and beliefs regarding the use of technology in patient care. *Computers, Informatics, Nursing*, 39 (11): 704–13. Available at: https://doi.otrg/10.1097/CIN.0000000000000791

Scammell, J. (2017) Person-centred care: what nurses can learn from the patient perspective. *British Journal of Nursing*, 26 (20):1133.

Scammell, J., Heaslip, V. and Crowley, E. (2016) Service user involvement in preregistration general nurse education: a systematic review. *Journal of Clinical Nursing*, 25 (1–2): 53–69.

Simms, D. (2020). Peer responses to trans youth tweeting about self-harm and suicidality. *Creative Nursing*, 26 (2): 135–42. Available at: https://doi.org/10.1891/CRNR-D-19-00089 (accessed 24 November 2022).

Smart, W. (2018) *Lessons learned review of the WannaCry Ransomware Cyber Attack*. NHS England. Available at: www.england.nhs.uk/wp-content/uploads/2018/02/lessons-learned-review-wannacry-ransomware-cyber-attack-cio-review.pdf (accessed 24 November 2022).

Suarez-Lledo, V. and Alvarez-Galvez, J. (2021) Prevalence of health misinformation on social media: systematic review. *Journal of Medical Internet Research*, 23 (1): e17187. Available at: https://doi.org/10.2196/17187 (accessed 24 November 2022).

Tan S.S.-L. and Goonawardene, N. (2017) Internet health information seeking and the patient–physician relationship: a systematic review. *Journal of Medical Internet Research*, 19: e9. Available at: https://doi.org/10.2196/jmir.5729 (accessed 24 November 2022).

Tapuria, A., Porat, T., Kalra, D., Dsouza, G., Xiaohui, S. and Curcin, V. (2021) Impact of patient access to their electronic health record: systematic review. *Informatics for Health and Social Care*, 46 (2): 192–204. Available at: https://doi.org/10.1080/17538157.2021.1 879810 (accessed 24 November 2024).

Topol Review (2019) *Preparing the Healthcare Workforce to Deliver the Digital Future.* Health Education England.

Towle, A., Bainbridge, L., Godolphin, W., Katz, A., Kline, C., Lown, B., . . . and Thistlethwaite, J. (2010) Active patient involvement in the education of health professionals. *Medical Education*, 44 (1): 64–74.

Tsou, A.Y., Lehmann, C.U., Michel, J., Solomon, R., Possanza, L. and Gandhi, T. (2017) Safe practices for copy and paste in the EHR. Systematic review, recommendations, and novel model for health IT collaboration. *Applied Clinical Informatics*, 8 (1): 12–34. Available at: https://doi.org/10.4338/ACI-2016-09-R-0150 (accessed 24 November 2022).

Tuman, M. (1992) *Word Perfect: Literacy in the Computer Age.* Pittsburgh, PA: University of Pittsburgh Press.

Vaillancourt, T., Faris, R. and Mishna, F. (2016) Cyberbullying in children and youth: implications for health and clinical practice. *Canadian Journal of Psychiatry*, 62 (6): 368–73. Available at: https://dx.doi.org/10.1177%2F0706743716684791 (accessed 24 November 2022).

Valenza, J.K., Boyer, B.L. and Curtis, D. (2014) Curation outside the library world. *Library Technology Reports*, 50 (7): 51.

van Houwelingen, C., Moerman, A., Ettema, R., Kort, H. and ten Cate, O. (2016) Competencies required for nursing telehealth activities: a Delphi-study. *Nurse Education Today*, 39: 50–62. Available at: https://doi.org/10.1016/j.nedt.2015.12.025 (accessed 24 November 2022).

van Laar, E., van Deursen, A., van Dijk, J. and de Haan, J. (2020) Determinants of 21st-century skills and 21st-century digital skills for workers: a systematic literature review. *SAGE Open*, 10 (1). Available at: https://doi.org/10.1177/2158244019900176 (accessed 24 November 2022).

Vasilica, C. (2015) Impact of using social media to increase patient information provision, networking and communication [PhD thesis]. *University of Salford*. Available at: https://usir.salford.ac.uk/id/eprint/38035/1/Cristina%20Vasilica%20ethesis%2023.6.15.pdf (accessed 24 November 2022).

Vasilica, C.M., Brettle, A. and Ormandy, P. (2020) A co-designed social media intervention to satisfy information needs and improve outcomes of patients with chronic kidney disease: longitudinal study. *JMIR Formative Research.* 4 (1). Available at: https://doi.org/10.2196%2F13207 (accessed 24 November 2022).

Vasilica, C.M., Garwood-Cross, L., Finnigan, R., Bashford, T., O'Kane, P. and Ormandy, P. (2021) Participating in CaMKIN: impact on patients. Available at: https://usir.salford.ac.uk/id/eprint/61117/1/Participating%20In%20CaMKIN%20Report%20v1.pdf (accessed 24 November 2022).

Warren, L.R., Clarke, J., Arora, S. and Darzi, A. (2019) Improving data sharing between acute hospitals in England: an overview of health record system distribution and retrospective observational analysis of inter-hospital transitions of care. *BMJ Open*, 9 (12). Available at: https://doi.org/10.1136/bmjopen-2019-031637 (accessed 24 November 2022).

Warrington, D.J., Shortis, E.J. and Whittaker, P.J. (2001) Are wearable devices effective for preventing and detecting falls: an umbrella review (a review of systematic reviews). *BMC Public Health*, 21 (1): 2091. Available at: https://doi.org/10.1186/s12889-021-12169-7 (accessed 24 November 2022).

Weiner, J.P., Kfuri, T., Chan, K., and Fowles, J.B. (2007). "e-Iatrogenesis": the most critical unintended consequence of CPOE and other HIT. *Journal of the American Medical Informatics Association*, 14 (3): 387–9. Available at: https://doi.org/10.1197/jamia.M2338 (accessed 24 November 2022).

Wheeler, A. J., Scahill, S., Hopcroft, D. and Stapleton, H. (2018) Reducing medication errors at transitions of care is everyone's business. *Australian Prescriber*, 41 (3): 73. Available at: https://doi.org/10.18773%2Faustprescr.2018.021

Williams, I., Allen, K. and Plahe, G. (2019) Restricted capital spending in the English NHS: a qualitative enquiry and analysis of implication. University of Birmingham: The Health Foundation.

Wilson, C., Ormandy, P., Vasilica, C. and Ali, S. (2016) '*e-Health diaries for people at end-of-life : "a crutch to lean on"*', in HIMS'16 : the 2016 International Conference on Health Informatics and Medical Systems, 25–8 July, Monte Carlo Resort, Las Vegas, NV, pp. 89–95.

Wong D.K.-K. and Cheung M.-K. (2019) Online health information seeking and eHealth literacy among patients attending a primary care clinic in Hong Kong: a cross-sectional survey. *Journal of Medical Internet Research*, 21. Available at: https://doi.org/10.2196/10831 (accessed 24 November 2022).

Woods, S.S., Schwartz, E., Tuepker, A., Press, N.A., Nazi, K.M., Turvey, C.L. and Nichol, W.P. (2013) Patient experiences with full electronic access to health records and clinical notes through the My HealtheVet Personal Health Record Pilot: qualitative study. *Journal of Medical Internet Research*, 15 (3). Available at: https://doi.org/10.2196/jmir.2356

World Health Organization (2011) *mHealth: New Horizons for Health through Mobile Technologies: Second Global Survey on eHealth*. Geneva: World Health Organization.

World Health Organization (2021) Infodemic. Available at: www.who.int/health-topics/infodemic#tab=tab_1

Zhang, J. and Cui, Q. (2018) Collaborative learning in higher nursing education: a systematic review. *Journal of Professional Nursing*, 34 (5): 378–88. Available at: https://doi.org/10.1016/j.profnurs.2018.07.00

Ziebland, S., Hyde, E. and Powell, J. (2021) Power, paradox and pessimism: on the unintended consequences of digital health technologies in primary care. *Social Science & Medicine*. Available at: https://doi.org/10.1016/j.socscimed.2021.114419 (accessed 24 November 2022).

Zucco, R., Lavano, F., Anfosso, R., Bianco, A., Pileggi, C. and Pavia, M. (2018) Internet and social media use for antibiotic-related information seeking: findings from a survey among adult population in Italy. *International Journal of Medical Informatics*, 111: 131–9. Available at: https://doi.org/10.1016/j.ijmedinf.2017.12.005 (accessed 24 November 2022).

Index